THE KEYNES PRESS

THE
GREAT MALARIA PROBLEM
AND ITS SOLUTION

Inscribed
To the People of SWEDEN
and to the memory of
ALFRED NOBEL

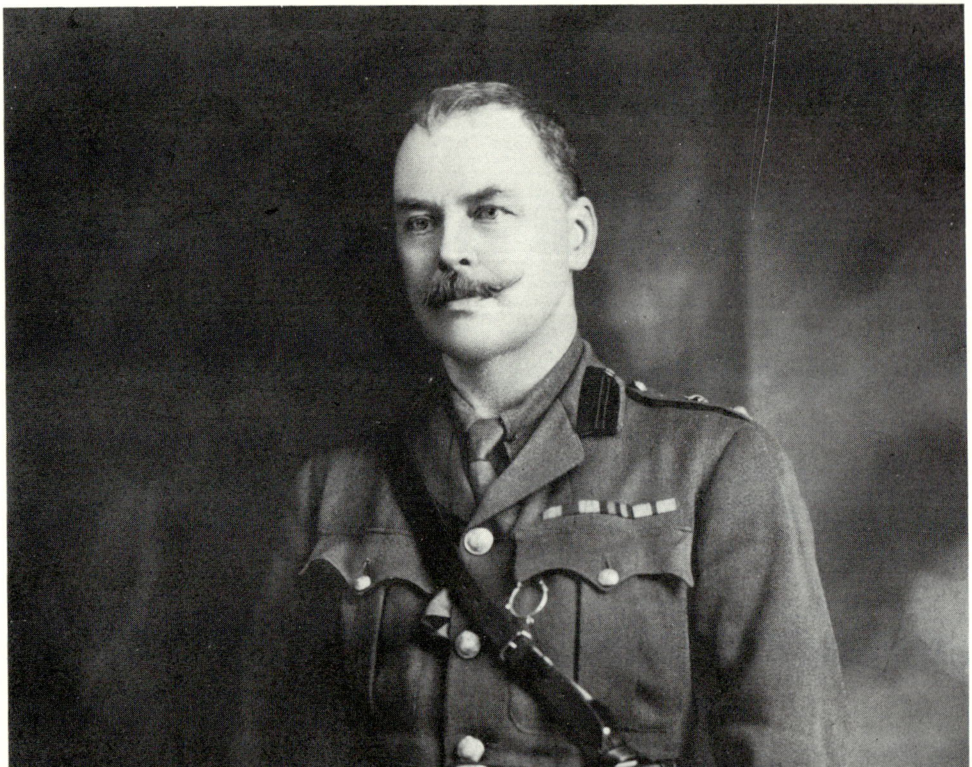

Ronald Ross.

The Great Malaria Problem and its Solution

FROM THE *MEMOIRS* OF

RONALD ROSS

WITH AN INTRODUCTION BY L J BRUCE-CHWATT

THE KEYNES PRESS
BRITISH MEDICAL ASSOCIATION

ISBN 0 7279 0172 9

First published as Part II of *Memoirs*
in 1923 by John Murray.
Published in 1988 by the Keynes Press
BMA House, Tavistock Square, London.

Made and printed in Great Britain by
Cambridge University Press

Contents

List of Plates

Preface

The solution of the malaria problem has been called the most dramatic episode in the history of medicine, and the facts when disclosed were certainly among the most wonderful in natural history; but the story has often been very inaccurately reported. Twenty years have elapsed since I first proposed to publish it in detail for medical readers—that is, with the correspondence and other matter now contained in this volume; but my numerous malaria expeditions, and then the compilation of my textbook on the prevention of malaria, and lastly the war interfered with the project.

The book is now complete, but I have decided to address it not only to medical men but to the general reader, in the form of my memoirs. There are several good reasons for this. In the first place it is hoped that the work will be of some practical use as regards the reduction of one of the most widespread of diseases. Now this is a matter which is always ultimately in the hands of laymen—it is they, not the doctors, who rule the world. Hitherto the matter has been left almost entirely to the medical profession, which, however, has failed to carry my scheme of 1899 to its logical conclusion, largely because it is allowed little influence in the world's counsels. Nothing, I am convinced, will really be done in this direction until those who govern us take the trouble to understand the subject. The only way to persuade them is to put the whole matter completely before them from my own point of view. In other words, the book is an appeal to Caesar; and I hope that he will deign to consider it.

But it has another object. A witty friend of mine once remarked that the world thinks of the man of science as one who pulls out his watch and exclaims, "Ha! half an hour to spare before dinner: I will just step down to my laboratory and make a discovery." Who but men of science themselves are to blame for such a misconception? Out of the many memoirs which fill our libraries few recount the labours of investigators, even of those who seek to solve the secrets of the great maladies which annually destroy millions of us—surely a matter of interest to everyone. Our books of science are records of results rather than of that sacred passion for discovery which leads to them. Yet many discoveries have really been the climax of an intense drama—full of hopes and despairs, visions seen in darkness, many failures, and a final triumph—in which the protagonists are man and nature and the issue a decision for all the ages. I trust, then, that this book at least will give a frank and accurate picture of one investigation, of the difficulties which attended it, and of the manner in which the world received and used, or did not use, the result.

In writing it I have seldom trusted to memory alone but have verified most of the details from the mass of documents—generally scribbled in the heat of action—which I possess. The book contains some criticisms which are required in the interests of human life or of science—it might usefully have contained more—but I have usually left the facts themselves to do the talking. Even for most of the misdoings mentioned here I must beg for the charity of humour because they were really due less to individuals than to that large and cheerful national indifference to all intellectual effort which our fathers called Philistinism. When this spirit applied merely to learning, art, and the more sidereal sciences it may perhaps be only lightly satirised; but what is to be said for it when it applies to matters of life and health of whole nations? Allied to it is that administrative barbarism which allows, for instance, a regiment to become infected with malaria because the officials cannot agree as to who shall hang the bed-nets; or which permits death-dealing street-puddles to remain in the midst of crowded and suffering cities for years after the danger of them has been fully demonstrated to all.

There is nothing, I hope, in these pages which the lay reader cannot easily understand; if there be, let him pass it over and proceed! We have, I fear, too much of the "first person singular" (besides many other faults), but I cannot trouble to correct this now; and, lastly, some events which might have found place in the final chapter have been resigned to the eloquence of silence.

I pray that the book will prove to be something more than a medical tale. Perhaps the kindly reader will perceive that when my malaria work was commenced 30 years ago as a self-imposed duty I had many ambitions closer to myself than it was. Indeed it was these ambitions which led to the malaria work as an episode, not always agreeable, in my life. They had given me, together with other pleasures, the philosophy of Epicurus, Lucretius, Comte, and Spencer; and I make my boast—among many other bravadoes—that I am one of the few among these masters' disciples who have attempted to bring their teaching to fruition!

For the rest, the world is worth living in: my complaints are mostly for others, not myself; for science; and for human life: and I have few misfortunes to boast about. If happiness had no history this book would not have been indited; and I now have the pleasure of ending it exactly a quarter of a century after that memorable day which occasioned it.

41 Buckingham Palace Mansions, RONALD ROSS.
London, S.W.1.
20 *August*, 1922.

Introduction

Of all the discoveries in medical science in the nineteenth century, few have been as dramatic as those revealing the nature of malarial fevers, the life cycles of the parasites concerned, their mode of transmission, and the possibilities of their control.

The introduction in the seventeenth century of the Peruvian bark (or Cinchona) from the New World was a major event as it brought into use a remarkable and specific remedy for intermittent fevers or agues. But the true cause of malaria was not known for another 250 years despite the rapid progress of the pasteurian era. Some erroneous observations of bacterial pathogens seemingly involved in malaria delayed scientific advance.

The first parting of the clouds came in 1880 when the French Army doctor Alphonse Laveran, while observing under a microscope a drop of blood from a febrile patient, saw vacuolated pigmented bodies in the erythrocytes and the lashing movements of the parasite's "flagellum." This discovery was received with scepticism, but after Laveran showed his preparations in Rome to a group of distinguished Italian parasitologists all of them became convinced. Within the next three years Camillo Golgi and others described three species of malarial plasmodia; they also showed their cyclical development and explained the relation of the periodicity of febrile attacks to the stages of growth of the parasites in the blood.

Nevertheless, for nearly 20 years after Laveran's discovery the mode of transmission of human plasmodia was still a mystery, although similar parasites of birds were discovered by Danilewsky. Many improvements of microscopical techniques were introduced by other Russian workers, while the American MacCallum explained the phenomenon of exflagellation first observed by Laveran.

Patrick Manson, the "father of tropical medicine," now enters into the story because of his fundamental discovery, made in China in 1878, of the mosquito transmission of filariasis. Other discoveries, of the role of ticks in the transmission of piroplasmosis (babesiosis) and of tsetse flies in African sleeping sickness, formed a background to Manson's conviction of mosquito involvement in malaria transmission, although no one suspected the true mechanism.

The dramatis persona who first revealed the complex development of malarial plasmodia in the mosquito was Ronald Ross, one of the most impressive and colourful individuals in the history of tropical medicine.

Ronald Ross was born at Almora, a hill station in the Kumaon Hills of India, on 13 May 1857, the eldest of the 10 children of General Sir Campbell Claye Grant Ross, of the Indian Army, and his wife, Matilda Charlotte Elderton. At the age of 8 Ross was sent to England for his education, first at a small school at Ryde and then at a boarding school at Springhill, near Southampton, where he remained until the age of 16. On leaving school he wanted to be a writer or artist but deferred to his father's wishes and in 1874 became a medical student at St Bartholomew's Hospital, London. He obtained his MRCS in 1879 and the licence of the Society of Apothecaries in 1881, went to sea for a year as a ship's surgeon, and then entered the Indian Medical Service. He arrived at Bombay and for some time was attached to various Madras regiments or to provincial military hospitals.

From September 1882 to August 1884 Ross was at Madras or on the move: he brought a detachment of Madras Pioneers from Quetta, he was posted with detachments of Indian troops to the Andamans, and from May 1885 to May 1886 he was in Burma. Having often enough time and leisure to follow his own pursuits, he studied with characteristic intensity the world's poets and the classics, took up Italian, French, and German, wrote poems, music, dramas, and novels, and became deeply interested in mathematics, which in later life entered into many of his works on malaria. In 1888 he left Madras for his first leave in England, where in 1889 he married Rosa Bessie Bloxam. During these years Ross appears as a capable young officer leading an intensely social and intellectual life, adopting various outdoor pursuits with enthusiasm, and writing his first romantic novel, *The Child of Ocean*.

In the summer of 1889 he took the diploma in public health in London and studied bacteriology under Professor E Klein. He had at that time no special interest in malaria, although he was deeply moved by the great misery and widespread sickness seen in rural India and expressed it in his poetry. In 1894 Ross once again came to England on leave. It was then that he was introduced to Sir Patrick Manson. Henceforth, the association of the older, already famous man with the young medical officer was to be a close and moving scientific partnership evidenced by 155 letters exchanged between them over the next four years.

In 1895 Ross won the triennial Parkes Memorial Prize for an essay on malaria. The next year he returned to India fired with the ambition to solve the problem of the transmission of this disease. But despite many efforts nothing that he tried seemed to solve the mystery. Finally, after many disappointments, he saw on 20 August 1897 the first sign of the success that had so far eluded him. He noticed on that day the characteristic pigmented "coccidia" (oocysts) of the malaria parasite in the stomach of an uncommon kind of "dapple-winged" mosquito (probably *Anopheles stephensi*) previously fed on a malarious patient. It was, however, not until June of the following year (1898), after he had taken up the study of Proteosoma, a genus of parasites causing bird malaria, that Ross found in other mosquitoes the same pigmented cysts and also further stages of their development, the "germinal rods" (sporozoites), in the salivary glands. Thus it became clear that malaria was an infection transmitted by the bites of mosquitoes.

On 28 July 1898 Manson announced Ross's discovery at the Edinburgh meeting of the British Medical Association; the whole astounding cycle of development of the malaria parasite was demonstrated for bird malaria and hence by analogy also for malaria of man. A convincing proof of the latter was provided in November 1898 by Grassi and his group in Rome.

In February 1899 Ross left India, having been invited by the Liverpool School of Tropical Medicine to take up the position of lecturer (later, 1902–12, professor) in tropical medicine; in July he retired from the Indian Medical Service. His mind was now turned almost wholly to the application of his discovery to the "extirpation" of malaria from the tropics by the destruction of the aquatic stages of anopheles mosquitoes. Several expeditions to West Africa were undertaken with this aim. Success was not as great as had been expected, for although the method was logical enough, difficulties in carrying it out on a large scale were underestimated. Ross did not spare himself in trying to convince the authorities of the possibilities of malaria control and eventually lived to see his methods applied with increasing success in many parts of the world.

Within a few years of his major discovery honours of every kind were conferred upon Ross by scientific institutions of many countries. In 1901 he was elected fellow of the Royal Society, which awarded him the Royal Medal in 1909; in 1902 he was awarded the Nobel Prize for medicine; he was appointed CB in 1902, KCB in 1911, and KCMG in 1918. He also received honorary degrees from several universities. During 1912 he moved to London and became physician for tropical diseases at King's College Hospital, an appointment which he combined (1912–17) with the chair of tropical sanitation at Liverpool. From 1913 until his death he was editor of *Science Progress*. During the war of 1914–18 he was appointed consultant in malaria to the War Office with the rank of lieutenant colonel and later to the Ministry of Pensions. When in 1926 the Ross Institute and Hospital for Tropical Diseases at Putney Heath was founded in his honour by a public subscription amounting to £50 000 he became its first director.

Sir Ronald Ross's life had not been free of sorrows: his elder son was killed in France during the retreat from Mons and one of his daughters died in childbirth. In 1927 he suffered a stroke, which left him partly paralysed. The death of Lady Ross in 1931 was a heavy blow, under which he slowly sank. He came to live at the Ross Institute, but his weakness increased almost daily. Waking after a long sleep on 16 September 1932 he suddenly said: "I shall find out things, yes, yes!" These were his last words. He was buried next to his wife at Putney Vale Cemetery, Roehampton.

In January 1934 the Ross Institute was incorporated into the London School of Hygiene and Tropical Medicine.

Ross's *Memoirs* are in many ways one of the most candid and revealing autobiographies that has ever been written by a famous medical man responsible for a major biological discovery. The book is of exceptional interest as, in addition to giving a complete and vivid account of his life and work, it shows the complexity of the author's nature and reveals a passionate defence of his acts and beliefs. Published in 1923 by John Murray, London, the book was awarded a year later the James Tait Black Memorial Prize for the best biography of 1923, the prize for the best novel going to Arnold Bennett for *Riceyman's Steps*. The present text comprises chapters VIII to XVIII of the original edition and tells the full story of the heroic period in Ross's life, from the origin of a scientific concept through the fumbling and thorny path of investigation to the climax of an intense human drama and final triumph.

On reading some of these pages one realises that most of Ross's work in India had been done under great difficulties and often against the opposition and obstacles of officialdom. Many letters exchanged between Manson and Ross are given in full and form the cream of the narrative. The present edition omits the scientifically less important and, to the general reader, less interesting period from 1900 onwards, dominated in the original book by Ross's intemperate attack on the "Roman brigandage" and Grassi's alleged dishonesty in attributing to himself the wisdom and the glory of the great discovery, to which he refers on page 224 in the last chapter of the present volume. The bitter personal controversy between Ross and Grassi presents one of the less edifying aspects of this dispute. Accusations coming from Ross against Grassi were so sharp that the first publisher of Ross's *Memoirs* feared they might be libellous, but Ross pleaded justification.

Ross's contributions to medicine during the later part of his life, although less spectacular, bear marks of his intellectual greatness. He was one of the first to lay the foundation of studies of communities exposed to malaria; the first to introduce the concept of malariometry as an epidemiological and diagnostic tool; the first to publish an account of the use of the "thick film" technique in blood microscopy.

The true sweep of Ross's original and fertile mind was revealed to all of us not long ago when the concept of malaria eradication was being elaborated during the halcyon days of the 1950s. His pioneering mathematical treatment of the complex phenomenon of malaria transmission was based on the "theory of happenings" described in the "*a priori* pathometry." Ross showed that the amount of malaria in an area tends towards a fixed limit determined by the interplay of the main factors involved, so that when the vector density is below a threshold level the disease tends to disappear. Detailed quantitative studies of malaria in the community were published by Ross in 1911; these formed a cornerstone for further work by a few other authors but were greatly expanded 30 years ago by Macdonald in Britain and Moshkovsky in the USSR. Something of the use and beauty of mathematics may be perceived, even by the non-numerate, when they grasp the meaning of an equation that expresses the subtle equilibrium of a biological system, even if it oversimplifies the natural happenings. Much work in this field is still proceeding with regard to the transmission dynamics of malaria and schistosomiasis.

Ross had all the qualities of a genius and also certain not uncommon faults. In some of his writings there is much self assertion, if not vanity, which, combined with his pugnacious temperament, was the target of criticism. To the outside world Ross was the dour adversary, the challenger, the castigator; but those who knew him well praised his kindness and his defence of just causes. Thus Ross's courageous fight to restore the good name of Haffkine, wrongly accused by the government of India of incompetence for producing a plague vaccine allegedly contaminated with tetanus bacilli, was an act of selfless and spontaneous generosity which won him many hearts.

Some of Ross's writings are occasionally marred by his grumbling about his emoluments, his pension, or his unsuccessful petition to the Chancellor of the Exchequer for a substantial compensation of financial losses caused by his scientific work. But they reflect Ronald Ross's personality "warts and all" and do not diminish the stature of a fullblooded and frank man of genius setting out on a great scientific adventure. That this adventure is still far from the expected success, 100 years after the first glimmer of light, and that our conquest of malaria may not be achieved by the end of the twentieth century is a singularly poignant and humiliating thought.

A few stirring lines written 30 years ago, on the sixtieth anniversary of Ross's discovery, by John Masefield, the late Poet Laureate and one of Sir Ronald's closest friends, honour the memory of this great man and evoke his unconquerable spirit:

Once on this August Day, an exiled man
Striving to read the hieroglyphics spelled
By changing speckles upon glass, beheld
A secret hidden since the world began.

The limitless instant of the joy laid bare
A force to alter life, a key, a clue,
Delaying Death and all his retinue;
Light showing as all answer to all prayer.

(*The Times*, 20 August 1957)

LEONARD JAN BRUCE-CHWATT
The Wellcome Tropical Institute
London, April 1986.

Glossary

A number of scientific terms used by Ross in the *Memoirs* are either those invented by him during his work in India or those generally used in scientific writings between 1890 and 1920 but obsolete now. Some of Ross's original suggestions concerning the terminology for the different stages of the development of malaria parasite can be found in the addenda to the book *The Prevention of Malaria*, 2nd edition, published by him in 1911, but few have been generally adopted.

The brief glossary given below follows much of the terminology of malaria as quoted by P C C Garnham in his authoritative *Malaria Parasites and other Haemosporidia* (1966).

Amoeba coli	A protozoon occurring in the intestine. The taxonomy of the genus is complex. It seems that Ross referred to the pathogenic form known as *Entamoeba histolytica*.
Anopheles costalis	*Anopheles gambiae* Giles.
Anopheles fuliginosus	*Anopheles annularis* V d Wulp.
Anopheles rossi	*Anopheles subpictus* Grassi.
Bioplasm	Cytoplasm.
Black spores	Dark banana shaped or round bodies, occasionally observed on the midgut wall of anopheles mosquitoes and probably caused by the secretion of chitin in response to an irritant.
Blasts	Synonym used by Ross for sporozoites.

Blastophore	Ross's term for the appearance of radial islets of cytoplasm ("sporoblasts") in a growing oocyst from which sporozoites are formed by budding (Plate I).
Blood plates	Blood platelets or thrombocytes.
Brindled (mosquitoes)	Brownish or tawny with streaks of other colour. (*Oxford English Dictionary*).
Cercomonas	A genus of flagellates present in faeces and in faecal cultures.
Chromatin	Nuclear body of cells that stains strongly with basic dyes.
Coccidia	Loose term for a group of protozoa of the order of Coccidia, parasites of the intestinal tract of animals and humans causing various forms of coccidiosis.
Coccidium	A term often loosely used by Ross in his letters and *Memoirs* (1923) for the oocyst stage of the development of malaria parasite in the gut of mosquitoes. He also applied this term to the gregarines. In reply to Nuttall's criticism Ross explained that these terms were provisional.
Coelome	Main body cavity of insects.
Crescents	Common term for gametocytes (sexual forms) of *Plasmodium falciparum* owing to their semilunar shape.
Crescent-sphere-flagella metamorphosis	Growth, maturation, and release of gametes (exflagellation) of male sexual stages of plasmodia.
Culex sylvestris	Probably *Aedes* (*Aedimorphus*) *vexans* Meigen.
Dacoits	Armed robber bands (Anglo-Indian (A-I)).
Dak bungalow	Travellers rest house (A-I).
Dappled-winged (mosquitoes)	Variegated with spots or patches of colour. (*Oxford English Dictionary*).
Dhooley bearer	Litter bearer (A-I).
Durwan	Porter or gatekeeper (A-I).
Exflagellation	The extrusion and liberation of microgametes by male gametocytes (microgametocytes).

Flagellates	Loose term for protozoa of the class of Mastigophora, which includes organisms that move by the help of specialized ectoplasmic structures, the flagella.
Flagellum (flagella)	A whip. An organ of locomotion of a number of protozoa. An early and common term (in plural) for microgametes released by male sexual cells (microgametocytes). Hence flagellulae, exflagellation, flagellated body, for the phenomenon of release of microgametes by the male gametocyte.
Gametids	Gametocytes, sexual forms of malaria parasites.
Germinal rods or threads	Ross's term for sporozoites, the final stage of development of the plasmodium in the mosquito. These are the infective forms of the malaria parasite released by the mature oocyst and invading the salivary glands of the mosquito.
Gregarines	Protozoa of the subclass of *Gregarinina*, intestinal parasites occurring in some insects, including mosquitoes.*
Grubs	Mosquito larvae.
Haemamoeba	Obsolete generic name for malaria parasites of primates but applicable to a subgenus of plasmodia in birds.
Haemomenas praecox	Obsolete name of *Plasmodium falciparum* causing the "aestivo-autumnal" (malignant tertian) fever.

* In 1895 Ross found parasites, which he believed to be some Coccidia, in the intestine of a *Stegomyia* (Aedes) mosquito. He then found them in the malpighian tubules and recognised them as encysted gregarines containing "psorosperms." These parasites were so common in larvae and adult mosquitoes in Secunderabad that Ross suspected them of representing a stage of the developing malaria parasite; however, he soon realised that they were of a different nature. The name *Gregarina culicis* given by Ross was changed to *Lankesteria culicis* in 1898. The remarkable cycle of development of this parasite related to the stages in the life of the insect was fully described in 1926 by Wenyon in his *Protozoology* (**2**: 1120–24). (See also Manson-Bahr P. The story of malaria—the drama and actors. *International Review of Tropical Medicine* Vol 2, Lincicome D R, ed. Academic Press, New York and London, 1963: 329–390.)

Haematozoin	Malaria pigment produced by the digestion of blood by the parasites. Haèmozoin is the correct term. Melanin is a wrong and obsolete term.
Haematids	Erythrocytes, red blood cells.
Haustellation	The process of sucking.
Imago	Adult mosquito, after emergence from the pupal case.
Karyokinesis	Mitosis, the process in which the nucleus divides.
Laveranity	Colloquial reference to Laveran's discovery of malaria parasite and its mosquito transmission.
Leukids	Leucocytes, white blood cells.
Malariated or malarialised	Infected by malaria parasites.
Malpighian tubules	Tubular glands connected with hind gut of insects. Their function is excretory.
Mere	Term used for a division of whole cell. Hence merozoite: product of division of a blood schizont (or of a tissue schizont).
Merozoite	Product of segmentation of erythrocytic and exo-erythrocytic schizonts.
Metaxeny	Change of hosts in succeeding generations of parasites.
Microsporidia	Protozoan organisms of the order Microsporidia, parasites of mammals, insects, crustacean, fish, and reptiles transmitted by spores.
Murrain	Infectious disease of unknown origin, often in cattle, imprecise term. (*Oxford English Dictionary*).
Nagana	Trypanosomal disease of cattle in tropical Africa, transmitted by tsetse flies.
Nosema	Genus of microsporidia causing disease of insects.
Oocyst	An encysted zygote in the mosquito stomach.

Panoplites	Former name of the mosquito genus *Mansonia*.
Piroplasma	Former name for the genus *Babesia*, parasites of cattle, sheep, horses, dogs, and occasionally humans, which invade blood corpuscles and cause specific diseases (piroplasmosis or babesiosis).
Polar bodies	Small round bodies at the edge of a mature female gametocyte (macro-gametocyte), formerly believed to be due to the reduction division of the nucleus; now known to represent part of the membrane of the erythrocyte after the escape of the macrogamete (Plate I).
Proteosoma relicta	This avian malaria parasite, the sporogonic development of which was demonstrated by Ross in 1897, is *Plasmodium* (*Haemamoeba*) *relictum*. The former name Halteridium was a synonym of *Haemo-proteus* of avian parasites in birds—for example, *H columbae* of pigeons.
Protospore	Ross's synonym for sporozoite.
Psorosperms (or pseudonav-icellae	Encysted forms of *Lankesteria culcis* found in the bodies of mosquitoes. Both Manson and Ross believed at first that they represented some stage of the development of malaria parasites, and Ross carried out a few experiments in humans (including himself) in 1895 (see footnote to page xix).
Schizont	Asexual parasite after the division of the nucleus. Hence schizogony.
Sperms or spermatozoa	Ross's occasional term for flagella (male gametes).
Spore	Single celled or multicelled reproductive body that becomes detached from the parent and gives rise, directly or in-directly, to a new individual. Occurring in plants, bacteria, and protozoa. Ross used this term rather freely for the

	trophozoites in the red blood cells and for the daughter cells (merozoites) formed by the segmenting schizont (Plate I).
Sporocytes	Obsolete name for merozoites, products of the division and multiplication of mature erythrocytic schizonts (schizogony).
Sporogony	Process of development of the malaria parasite occurring in the mosquito after the union of male and female gametes and ending with the formation of sporozoites.
Sporulation	The process of spore formation.
Stegomyia calopus	Former name of *Aedes aegypti*, a mosquito responsible for transmission of yellow fever and other viral diseases.
Terai	A large stretch of marshy or overgrown land with underwood or tangled vegetation (A-I).
Vermicule	Also "travelling vermicule," a motile stage of the zygote, before the formation of the oocyst on the gut of the mosquito.
Undulant fever	Also called Malta fever, a disease now known as brucellosis, caused by *Brucella melitensis* and other species of this bacterium in humans and also (*B abortus*) in cattle, swine, sheep, goats, and horses.
Zygote	The product of the union of male and female gametes.

I am grateful to Professor P C C Garnham, FRS, for his comments on this glossary.

1

The Problem

As four years of my life were devoted almost entirely to investigations on malaria I must make an effort to describe the subject in language suitable to the lay reader. It is the main object of this book to interest him in the matter. The lay reader rules the world. We doctors are only helots. We advise, he snubs us; we advise again and perhaps some day he listens to us! But I hope also to win the suffrage of men of science by an accurate history of the events.

Malarial fever is the most common of infective diseases almost throughout the tropics and occurs during the summer even in temperate climates. In the tropics it causes roughly about one third of all the attendances at hospitals and about one third of the entire population suffers from it every year. Although only about one case in several hundreds dies of it, yet the prevalence of the disease is so enormous that the total aggregate of the deaths directly due to it, and still more indirectly due to it, is colossal. Thus it has been officially estimated that in India alone something like 1 300 000 deaths were caused by it in years during which it was not exceptionally prevalent; and at the end of last century out of about 300 000 men in the army in India, 100 000 were admitted into hospital every year for malaria. Similar statistics are given for almost all hot countries except Egypt and some other isolated tracts; in Greece and round Rome the disease is a curse; and it has prevailed in Europe as far north as Holland, England (in 1917 and 1918), and Sweden. In addition to the actual frequency of infection most cases tend to relapse even for years after the original attack; and lastly malaria has a great political influence because it haunts especially the most fertile and well watered parts of the earth. Probably malaria has done more than anything else to prevent the settlement and civilisation of the vast tropical areas which would otherwise be most suitable for the human race. All knowledge connected with malaria is therefore of the very first practical importance for mankind in general.

The disease itself is an intermittent fever—that is, a fever characterised by regular recurrences every day or every two or three days (called quotidian, tertian, and quartan fever respectively). The recurrences generally begin about midday, often with severe chills and shivering (rigor or ague attack), succeeded by high temperature reaching 105 ° F or more. This fever continues for variable periods up to 20 hours or more and then abates with profuse sweating. Sometimes, however, in quotidian or even in tertian fever a second attack commences before the preceding one has quite abated, when we have what is called a remittent fever. In badly treated cases these recurrences may continue for weeks and sometimes, with intervals of comparative quiescence, for years. I remember that my father had a typical relapse of malaria just as we were sitting down to lunch one day in 1888, eight years after he had left India, and relapses after much longer periods are known to occur. On the other hand many cases recover completely after the first few attacks and most cases recover naturally about the third, fourth, or fifth years of infection. In 1900 Robert Koch discovered that most native children in malarious areas in the tropics are infected shortly after birth and remain infected, or are reinfected over and over again, until they reach about 15 years of age, when they appear to throw off the infection and become partially immune. A single attack of the fever causes considerable anaemia and when the attacks recur frequently the patient may become very anaemic and weak, though he tends to rally during the periods of quiescence. The large gland called the spleen, which is situated just above the lower edge of the ribs of the left side, rapidly increases in size when the attacks are numerous (if no quinine be given) and sometimes becomes extremely large (splenomegaly). The disease is usually what is called a benign one, but fatal cases sometimes occur early in the infection in certain dangerous varieties called pernicious attacks, among which the famous blackwater fever is the most common cause of death. Probably early deaths from malaria are the principal cause of child mortality in tropical countries, but even when patients do not die from the disease they may be kept for years in a weak state and unable to work and may be carried off at the beginning of the cold season by dysentery or pneumonia. Of course the general use of the specific remedy, quinine, modifies much the progress of the illness, which must have been a very serious matter in the days before quinine was discovered. During the war [of 1914–18] a number of cases were accidentally infected with malaria and were not treated by quinine early enough owing to the fact that the infection was not discovered in time and a large proportion of these men died—showing the potential severity of the disease, especially in the form called malignant tertian.

Necessarily all nations living in warm countries are only too well acquainted with malaria, and the ancient Greeks and Romans were no exception to this rule. After I visited Greece in 1906 I enunciated the hypothesis that malaria may have entered that country for the first time during the earliest ages, just as it entered Mauritius in 1866 in the memory of people now living[1]; and subsequently Mr W H S Jones of Cambridge gave us a laborious and exhaustive study on the subject made in the light of our present knowledge.[2] There are few references to malaria in the earliest literature but many in later writings. For a summary of this interesting theme see my book *The Prevention of Malaria*.[3]

It is well known that the ancients recognised the quartan, tertian, quotidian, and semitertian (probably malignant tertian) varieties of malaria and many of its accidents and that they were acquainted with its seasonal and local variability and, above all, with its frequent prevalence near marshes. This last point is most germane to our present part of the subject.

Thus Strabo (1st century BC) says that Alexandria, in spite of its site, was free from marsh fever (paludism) even in his time. "It is to be inferred from this," Mr Jones says, "that damp places were generally known to be unhealthy, so that exceptions to the rule were noticed by observers as remarkable phenomena."

For ancient Italy we have a similar story—namely, that references to paludism are scanty in the earlier writers but very abundant in the later ones. Many areas round Rome, now scarcely habitable, were the homes of great and prosperous peoples in the prehistoric period and later were full of the country villas of rich Romans.

Of course the Roman writers, both medical and non-medical, were acquainted with the leading facts about paludism mentioned above. There are also several passages referring to mosquito nets, called *conopeum* by the Romans after the Greeks (our word canopy). Herodotus first noted with surprise the use of them in Egypt and they are referred to later by Varro (*De re rustica*, 2, 10, 8), Horace (*Epodes*, 1, 16), Propertius (3, 11, 45), Juvenal (6, 80), and Paulus Silentiarius (*Anthologia palatina*).

Little was added to our knowledge during the next 1500 years; but about 1640 the inestimable boon of cinchona bark was introduced into Europe. The Countess d'El Cinchon, wife of the Viceroy of Peru, had been cured of fever by means of it in that country, where it had been discovered by the Indians near Loxa (?), and she was wise enough to send it home to Europe. The use of it, after many checks, gradually spread and in 1820 Pelletier and Caventou extracted the alkaloid quinine from it. But the discovery of this specific has not only proved to be a blessing for the treatment of untold millions of human beings but also enabled Morton (1697) and Torti (1753) to separate the malarial fevers, which are cured by it, from those upon which it has no influence and by this means to differentiate and study the symptoms of the former. Morton also recalled the old hypothesis of the marsh and this was amplified by Lancisi, who repeated the ancient sayings of Varro[4] and Palladius[5] in greater detail in his book *De noxiis paludum effluviis*.[6] He stated that fevers disappear after drainage and attributed the poison either to inorganic or to organic emanations from the marsh. He studied mosquitoes and even (?) suggested inoculation by them as a possible means of infection—though he also thought that their larvae foul drinking water.

It is now apparent that the world had been gradually becoming aware during centuries of the paludic nature of malarial fever, not by direct experiment or even by investigation, but by a kind of subconscious experience based on public observations. In Italy especially, where of all civilised countries the disease was most prevalent, this process was most apparent. More than this, by similar general observation the good effect of assainment of marshes had become equally notorious there. Thus as early as 1667 Doni wrote a work called *De Restituenda Salubritate Agri Romani*; and references to a succession of works carried out on this principle, which I now call the principle of mosquito reduction, were given by Celli (1901). At the same time efforts were made by many observers, such as Morton, Lancisi, Lind, and Pringle, to explain the paludic connection and these resulted in the hypothesis of the "paludic miasma." This was supposed to be some kind of infecting emanation from stagnant water, either chemical or, as Lancisi suggested, organic; but in no cases, apparently, were experiments made to test the point. Later, when it was observed that malaria may sometimes occur where there is no marsh, the hypothesis of the paludic miasma was extended to become that of the "telluric miasma," according to which the poison exists not only in marshes but anywhere in suitable soil, from which it rises at night or when the soil is disturbed. This speculation, for it was nothing more, is not quite dead even yet, though the observation which originated it is easily explained otherwise. The word "malaria" (*mal'aria*, or bad air) is derived from it. Many writers attributed the disease to various marsh-growing vegetable organisms. In 1862 Salisbury in particular, after considerable study, blamed a kind of palmella [an alga]; and after 1878 a number of Italian workers, Lanzi and Terrigi, E Klebs, and C Tommasi-Crudeli, thought that they had actually incriminated certain fungi or bacteria which they said swarm in malarious places, occur in the blood, produce spores before each paroxysm of fever, and cause similar infection in animals. These findings were even confirmed by Marchiafava and other Italians but have now been completely discredited.

Meantime, however, other light had been thrown on the subject from various quarters. As long ago as 1846 Rasori made an extraordinary prediction on this subject. "For many years," he said, "I have held the opinion that the intermittent fevers are produced by parasites that cause the successive paroxysms of fever by their reproduction, which occurs periodically more or less rapidly according to their species"—and this has proved to be exactly true. But it was only speculation, and modern pathological science demanded strict microscopical and experimental evidence. I had the same idea about 1883.

In 1847 H Meckel discovered innumerable black granules in the blood of an insane patient[7] and the discovery was subsequently confirmed and amplified by other observers—the granules (Plate I) now being known under the name of the paludic pigment, melanin, or haematozoin (Sambon). For a long time they were thought to be due to a chemical action of the paludic miasma on the red cells of the blood. This, however, was discredited in 1878 when C Gerhardt proved that healthy persons can be infected by the inoculation of blood of patients suffering from paludism. His experiments were afterwards verified by many workers and demonstrate (apart from the subsequent microscopical discovery of the parasites) that the disease is not due to any gaseous emanation from marshes but is a true infection by some living virus.

Now came a great discovery. In 1878 A Laveran, a French army surgeon, commenced his studies of the subject at Bône in Algeria by following up the granules of pigment already referred to in the blood of living patients. He was struck by the fact that they were frequently contained within the red corpuscles in small cells possessing active amoeboid movements (Plate I, figs 2–4, 8–10); and finally,[8] on 6

November 1880 at Constantine, he detected the sperms (microgametes, flagella) issuing from the male cell (flagellated body, Plate I, fig 16). Though at the time he did not know the nature of this phenomenon, it convinced him that he was dealing with minute parasites which live in or on the human red corpuscles like maggots within nuts. In fact, the black granules are merely the excrementitious matter produced by the parasites from the substance of the red cells and retained within their bodies to be ultimately released in the tissues of the host.

I must next explain some points for the lay reader. The blood of an average adult consists of some fifteen million million little discs of yellow jelly called the red corpuscles floating in a fluid called the serum. About 3400 red corpuscles touching each other and lined up in a straight line would occupy one inch. When a droplet of blood is taken from the finger of a patient and spread between two surfaces of glass under the microscope these red corpuscles can easily be seen placed out flatly like plates on a table and Laveran now discovered that in malaria many of them contain a little pale circular patch without the yellow colour of the corpuscle. In fresh blood, however, these little patches can be seen to be constantly changing shape—that is, they possess amoeboid movement—and they can also be seen to contain one or more minute black particles of melanin. They appear to grow in size within the corpuscle and end by filling it up almost entirely, and then they contain a large number of melanin granules. When mature they break up into separate portions called spores (Plate I, fig 5) and then the corpuscle containing them breaks and the spores are liberated in the serum to infect fresh corpuscles (Plate I, fig 6). These are the asexual forms of the malaria parasite, which was subsequently named *Plasmodium*.

But in addition to these forms Laveran saw what were evidently bodies of the same class but not contained at all in corpuscles—that is, bodies full of melanin lying by themselves in the serum (Plate I, figs 11, 12). While watching one of these at Constantine in 1880 he saw, as I have said, the melanin granules become violently agitated and then observed that long filaments issued from the parent body and wriggled about violently as if attempting to escape from it (Plate I, fig 19). He thought that these filaments were flagella, like the flagella which enable many small organisms in water to move about; and the whole body with these so-called flagella attached became generally known under the name of the flagellate body. These bodies are now known to be not really flagellate bodies at all but the male sexual forms of the plasmodium, the filaments being sperms (Plate I, fig 21).

The whole history of the researches detailed in this book depends upon these sexual forms. Laveran was wrong in the role which he attributed to them; but that does not diminish the glory of his discovery, which has revolutionised medical science in the tropics. At that time, owing to the work of Pasteur, Koch, and others, many diseases were known to be due to vegetable parasites called bacteria etc; but Laveran's organism was evidently a minute *animal* parasite belonging to the most elementary class of animals called the single-celled animals or protozoa.

Laveran next showed that his parasites occur in cases of malaria but not in healthy persons. He could not, however, work out their life history completely; but in 1886 and subsequently C Golgi, who was favourably situated in Pavia for the work, showed clearly that the asexual parasites reproduce themselves by forming spores (as mentioned above—Plate I, figs 5, 6); that all these parasites in the body tend to produce the spores at about the same hour; and that it requires 72 hours for the quartan parasite to form its spores and 48 hours for the tertian parasite to do the same. He proved also that the attack of fever in the patient commences at the moment when the spores are liberated (just as Rasori had divined). This explains the difference between the quartan and the tertian fevers and Golgi showed further that the shapes and appearances of the organisms which cause quartan (*Plasmodium malariae*) and mild tertian fever (*Plasmodium vivax*) are different, so that the variety of parasite concerned can easily be detected at once under the microscope. A little later Canalis and Marchiafava and Celli discovered similar facts regarding the malignant parasites (*Plasmodium falciparum*, Plate I) and showed that they differ from the quartan and mild tertian parasites; and Marchiafava and Bignami suggested that they are of two varieties, the malignant tertian and the quotidian. In 1885 Danilewsky discovered similar parasites in birds and several other animals and subsequently Marchiafava, Celli, Bignami, Mannaberg, and others made many careful studies of the parasites and of their effects in human beings, Romanowsky found the proper way to stain them, and many observers verified these researches in various parts of the world, the literature amounting to some hundreds of publications. But up to 1894 no one had conceived the meaning of the sexual forms of plasmodia (Plate I, figs 10, 11, 12). That is where our work commences.

The question now arose—an all important question in connection with the prevention of the disease—how do these parasites manage to effect an entry into the blood of men and animals? Most observers, remembering that the disease often abounds in the neighbourhood of marshes, assumed at once that Laveran's parasites must be capable of living in a changed form in stagnant water and some actually sought them there. Thus Grassi and Calandruccio suggested that a free-living amoeba is really the external stage of the organism. On the other hand experiments to infect healthy persons by water from marshes, made by Marchiafava and Celli (1885), Marino (1890), and especially Agenore Zeri (1890), failed entirely.

But some other considerations should have been remembered by students of the subject but were not. These minute animal parasites of the blood were quite possibly subject to a common law governing many larger parasites, called the law of metaxeny or change-of-host. Until the beginning of the 18th century all parasites of men and animals were supposed, like other low forms of life, to be created in each host (that is, the animals containing the parasites) by "spontaneous generation." Very gradually the zoologists showed that these parasites, like other animals, develop solely from their own eggs. In 1790, however, Abildgaard made the remarkable discovery by experiment that a certain parasite not only develops from its own eggs but migrates from one host, a fish, into another host, a waterfowl, which feeds on the said fish. The law was further developed in 1841 and finally established for certain parasites by F Küchenmeister, physician to the Duke of Saxe Meiningen, in 1851–3. The famous German parasitologist R Leuckart established many new cases. An important one was that of *Filaria medinensis*, or guineaworm of man, which was found by Fedschenko sometime before 1869, at Leuckart's suggestion, to pass a stage of life in the little water-flea called *Cyclops*. In 1877 Patrick Manson in Amoy, China, showed that another filaria of man, *Filaria bancrofti* or *nocturna*, has a similar development in a mosquito.[9] This was the first time that metaxeny was found to occur with any parasite between men and mosquitoes; but Manson did not observe the development to a stage much more advanced than that observed by Fedschenko in cyclops (page 13).

All these examples of metaxeny were concerned only with the higher parasites, the helminths or worms. But the objects discovered by Laveran belong to a much lower class of animal; and though many organisms of this class were later discovered in various animals, yet up to 1889 not one of them had been proved to be metaxenous. Then, however, Theobald Smith and F L Kilborne in America showed[10] that the little parasite of Texas cattle fever called *Piroplasma bigeminum* is communicated by a tick, though they did not find the parasite actually living in the tick and therefore did not prove any alternate generation in them. Meantime, however, several diseases had been popularly connected with the bites of insects etc. Many travellers related that natives ascribe a peculiar sickness to the bites of another kind of tick and others said that the deadly nagana of cattle in parts of Africa is probably due to the bites of the tsetse fly—proved later by Bruce[11]; and it is now important to note that similar speculations connecting both yellow fever and malaria with mosquitoes had long been rife, though they were generally derided at the time and speedily forgotten.

I have already alluded to the curious utterances of Varro, Palladius, and Lancisi regarding insects and fever. Nuttall[12] gives statements by Lustig, Rübner, Koch, and myself to the effect that the peasantry in Italy, Tyrol, East Africa, and Assam seemed to have vague ideas of the same kind. Dr R H Kennan informed me that he had found an old ordinance of Freetown, Sierra Leone, dated 1812 in which the inhabitants (mostly freed slaves) are enjoined to keep the road in front of their plots in good condition in order to prevent the formation of "stagnant pools which generate disease and mosquitoes over the town." In 1848 Dr Josiah Nott, of Mobile, Alabama, appears to have stated that both yellow fever and malaria may be transmitted by mosquitoes and refers to the speculation as having been already advanced as regards malaria. In 1854, however, Louis Daniel Beauperthuy, a French medical man born in Guadeloupe in 1808, gave the hypothesis in greater detail.[13] As a "travelling naturalist" for the Paris Museum in Venezuela he studied both these diseases microscopically and concluded that they are produced by a venomous fluid injected under the skin by mosquitoes, like the poison injected by snakes. Marshes, he says, are dangerous because of the mosquitoes bred in them, not because of their effluvia. He surmised that several species of mosquito carry yellow fever but mentioned especially "the *Zancudo bobo* with legs striped with white"—probably *Stegomyia calopus*,* which we now know is really the agent. But he gives no proofs in support of his opinions, which were only speculations based upon general thought and observation or fancy.

In 1881 and subsequently Charles Finlay, of Havana, repeated a similar hypothesis, apparently independently of Nott and Beauperthuy.[14] His views, however, differ in an important particular. While Beauperthuy seemed to think that mosquitoes originally obtain the disease-giving poison from the marsh in which they breed (and apparently Lancisi believed the same), Finlay held (regarding yellow fever) that they obtain it from sick people. In other words, he thought

* J Guiteras says *not* (*Lancet*, 18 June 1910).

that the insects simply convey it from patients to healthy persons. The proboscis of a mosquito which bites a patient becomes contaminated by germs in his blood, the germs multiplying in the proboscis and then entering the blood of any person whom the mosquito bites next—just as bacteria may be carried on a soiled surgical instrument from one person to another. He thought that an insect which had only just bitten a patient could convey the virus but that the longer it lived after biting the patient the more the germs would multiply in its proboscis and the larger the dose given to the healthy person would be. He also considered that a mosquito with striped legs (*Stegomyia calopus*) is the agent of yellow fever. He records some experiments, but they must have been very doubtful since we know now that mosquitoes which have bitten a patient must live for no less than 12 days before they can infect a healthy person. Like Beauperthuy he rightly conjectured the species of mosquito which carried yellow fever and actually placed them in the hands of the men who ultimately solved the problem. He was acquainted with Manson's researches on the development of *Filaria bancrofti* in mosquitoes.

In 1883 Dr A F A King wrote an able paper on the subject[15] in which he gives no fewer than 19 reasons why mosquitoes are likely to carry paludism. These are: that both paludism and mosquitoes (*a*) are connected with marshes; (*b*) require a temperature of over 60 °F; (*c*) are checked at freezing point; (*d*) abound most near the equator and seacoasts; (*e*) have an affinity for dense foliage; (*f*) can be screened off by trees; (*g*) can be transported by winds; (*h*) are encouraged by turning the soil; (*i*) are affected by "bodies of water"; (*j*) are diminished by cultivation and settlement; (*k*) keep near the surface of the ground; (*l*) abound most after sundown; (*m*) and in the open; (*n*) are destroyed by fires; (*o*) are not so common in cities; (*p*) are most prevalent in autumn; (*q*) are arrested by mosquito nets; (*r*) affect infants (which are generally protected by nets) less than adults; and (*s*) attack whites more than other races. This was by far the best exposition yet given. Though arguments *d*, *m*, *n*, *r*, and *s* are not sound while arguments *e*, *f*, and *g* are very doubtful, and though the most cogent argument of all was not known to him, the cumulative effect of his careful and well arranged reasoning was very strong. Like Beauperthuy he held that the insects bring the poison from the marsh and inoculate it by their bites. He was acquainted with Manson's work but not with Laveran's. All these speculations were speedily lost sight of and were not resuscitated until my researches had cleared up the question.

About the same time Laveran[16] suggested the same idea [p 457] in a short sentence: "Do mosquitoes play the same role in paludism as in filariasis?" he said. "The thing is not impossible and we must note that mosquitoes abound in all marshy places."

Also about the same time, during his famous studies on cholera in India, R Koch had the same notion but he mentioned it only in his lectures to students [Nuttall[12] p 77, and Ross[17] p 73].

I now return to my personal narrative. Though it was certain that malarial fever is caused by parasites in the blood and though the disease had actually been communicated from man to man by the inoculation of the blood of infected persons, still in 1894 we did not even guess, much less know for certain, how these parasites manage to pass from the sick to the healthy *under natural conditions*. This was evidently an all important matter for tropical sanitation because without such knowledge it was impossible for us to construct any scientific basis for the prevention of the disease and therefore for saving a gigantic amount of misery in the world. It was my duty to attack the problem at this point. I call it here the Great Problem!

Though some savants had *suggested* that the mosquito carries the infection in some way, the world, even the medical world, remained sublimely ignorant of and indifferent to the matter and everyone held the old hypothesis mentioned on page 5 that, as its name implies, malaria is due to bad air from marshes. But I had long felt that this was not sufficient explanation and in my voyage to Burma in 1889 I saw cases which could scarcely be so explained and began to consider the matter very carefully. At this time the medical services in India were so badly organised that medical libraries did not even exist in the principal stations,* and while individual medical officers often did good clinical work, there was little investigation and almost no establishment for it and we British cheerfully lived up to our reputation of being an unscientific if not an unintellectual race. Even the great bacteriological discoveries of Pasteur and Koch were scarcely recognised, or were ridiculed, and Laveran's was almost unheard of. Apart from individual workers such as Vandyke Carter, Lewis, and Cunningham the services did not concern themselves much with medical investigation. Hence when I began to think about the cause of malaria I could get neither advice nor literature and at first fell into errors. To begin with, after my arrival in Bangalore in May 1890 I did some work on the hypothesis that these fevers might really be due to some kind of intestinal poisoning and published four papers on it.[18] I did not know that the French physician Broussais had

* I understand that this has not even yet been always remedied.

anticipated me in this—and we were both wrong. In 1892, however, several writers in India began to publish papers on Laveran's parasite, but unfortunately described not the plasmodium but a number of appearances in the blood which resemble it. The error was speedily detected by me and exposed in four more papers[19] and this, of course, led me (and others) to doubt whether Laveran's work was sound. By bad luck, though I searched innumerable specimens, I failed to find the plasmodium at all, partly because my technique was too beautiful and complicated! I did not see Vandyke Carter's genuine work till I was in England in 1894. Thus all my laborious studies during these years 1890–94, were ineffective, but the failures educated me and I had time to consider the subject very thoroughly and to become a competent microscopist. I had sent to England for Laveran's books in 1892 if I remember aright and I always subscribed to the *Indian Medical Gazette* and the *British Medical Journal*. Laveran's descriptions and drawings of the parasites were, as everyone admits, so poor that it was not surprising that few recognised his bodies at first from his writings. At any rate I failed to do so and therefore thought that his work was unsound or even a pretence.

On my arrival in England in March 1894 I went at once to Professor Kanthack, the pathologist at St Bartholomew's Hospital, who assured me that Laveran's discovery was sound and referred me to Dr Patrick Manson, then living in Queen Anne Street, Cavendish Square. I wrote to him at once and called on him on about 10 April 1894. Within a few minutes he showed me the Laveran's bodies which are technically called "crescents" in a stained specimen of malaria blood and I recognised at once that no such bodies exist in healthy blood. My doubts were now removed; and in a few days Manson demonstrated the other forms of the organisms to me in a patient lying at Charing Cross Hospital and also took me on several occasions, with great kindness, to the Seamen's Hospital (at the Royal Albert Dock in East London) and made me acquainted with translations of the illuminating monographs on malaria by Mannaberg and by Marchiafava and Bignami in Vol CL of the New Sydenham Society's publications. Subsequently the distinguished microscopist Dr H G Plimmer, FRS, told me that he had similarly demonstrated the bodies to Manson some time previously.

Dr Manson (afterwards Sir Patrick Manson, GCMG, FRS, MD) was then a good looking, rather tall man of 50 who had practised for some years in China, where he had done excellent medical and parasitological work on various skin diseases and also on the terrible deforming malady called elephantiasis. He had practically shown this to be due to the small worms which live in the lymphatics and the blood vessels and are called *Filaria bancrofti*. But more than this, either on his own initiative or on that of Bancroft, he had shown that the young of the parasites are sucked up with the blood of patients by mosquitoes (species then undetermined), in which insects they grow and develop to a considerable size.[9] He did not work out the whole life history of the filaria but thought that the insect dies after laying her eggs on water, when the parasites escape out of her dead body into the said water in which they are drunk up by healthy persons, who thus become infected. This life history, which he discovered in 1877, was very like that of *Filaria medinensis* in cyclops, discovered previously by the Russian naturalist Fedschenko, on Leuckart's suggestion, after 1858. Both life histories were incomplete, and Manson's conjecture that the filaria embryos return to water after living in the mosquito was wrong, for after my researches had shown that mosquitoes not only take the malaria parasite from infected persons but also inoculate them after a week or more into healthy persons (1898) James, Low, and others proved a similar procedure regarding *Filaria bancrofti*. I gather that Manson could scarcely have done much actual *experimental* work on the subject because he certainly instructed me that the insects live only from three to five days after feeding,* while the filariae are now known to require three weeks for development in mosquitoes. I gathered also from him that he had worked only with the insects caught in the godown in which his servant infected with *filariae* lived (see also Manson's article in Andrew Davidson's *Hygiene and Diseases of Warm Climates*, 1893, p 771, Edinburgh, Young J Pentland). But undoubtedly he observed the first stages of the parasite in his mosquitoes (probably a culex) and figures them correctly and the above facts do not detract from the very great merit of his work.

Manson had now retired from China since some years and had commenced practice in London. He treated me with the greatest kindness and I visited him often and learnt all he had to tell me. I do not remember having done malaria work in London during the summer of 1894 (and was in Switzerland for six weeks), but in November I called upon him again and found him just starting for the Seamen's Hospital. I went with him and remember distinctly that as we were walking along Oxford Street at about 2.30 pm he said to me: "Do you know, I have formed the theory that mosquitoes carry malaria just as they carry

* I showed in 1897 that mosquitoes, even in captivity, live much longer than five days (page 110) merely if they are fed frequently enough.

filariae." I replied at once that I had seen the same conjecture in one of Laveran's books.[16]

Manson then explained his cogent reasons for his belief. As I have said (page 9), others had previously suspected that malaria is carried by mosquitoes, but mostly on very inadequate grounds; and we did not even know of these writings at that time. Manson now added a new and stronger argument to those already mentioned. We knew the function of the *asexual* forms of the parasites but were ignorant of the functions of what were later proved to be the *sexual* forms—the so-called crescents and flagellate bodies (Plate I, figs 11–20). Shortly after blood containing these forms is drawn from a patient's finger the crescents swell up, become oval and then spherical, and lastly sometimes emit the long and actively motile filaments (Plate I, fig 19) which were then wrongly called flagella, and these may sometimes be seen under the microscope to break away from the parent cell and to wriggle about rapidly in the fluid of the blood (Plate I, fig 21). They had long been subjects of discussion. Some observers, chiefly of the Italian school, held that they represent only the dying struggles of the parasite; others, including Laveran and Danilewsky, thought that they are really living bodies and Mannaberg even suggested that they may be connected with the life history of the parasites outside the human body—though he did not explain how this could be. Manson now offered an explanation. He thought that when the mosquito sucks the blood these sexual forms enter its stomach and there, in a few minutes, emit their motile filaments just as they do under the microscope. The motile filaments, he thought, were flagellated spores which next pass through the walls of the mosquito's stomach and take up their abode in its tissues, where they must develop further into some unknown stage and then enter drinking water. Here he was wrong.

But I was immensely impressed with this argument and determined to test the hypothesis thoroughly on my return to India. A few weeks later Manson published a short article describing his hypothesis.[20] Of course we discussed the best procedure for me to follow and decided that I should work if possible with crescents (now known to be the sexual forms of *Plasmodium falciparum*). Manson described his technique with *Filaria bancrofti*, but as this was a very much larger parasite his experiences with it did not help me much with malaria. I tried to obtain works on mosquitoes but failed entirely—probably because, very unwisely, I did not inquire at the British Museum, a most unfortunate failure because there *were* some entomological papers on the subject; and I never even received Ficalbi's treatise which appeared next year.[21] I was also ignorant of the Romanowsky method of staining the malaria parasites, though this had been discovered some years previously. In fact I went forth very badly equipped for the fray.

Before leaving England in March 1895 I won (20 March) the Parkes Memorial (triennial) Prize offered at Netley Hospital to members of the medical services for the best essay on malaria.[22] It consisted of a gold medal and 75 guineas. I have just read, for the first time since it was written, my draft of the essay. It admits Laveran's parasite and Manson's induction, describes (with many photomicrographs) the natural appearances in the blood which were being mistaken for plasmodia, shows why I had failed to find the latter, and deals with the numerous fevers which were then confused with malaria. But the chief merit of the essay lay in its destructive analysis of textbook theories of aerial convection of the infection from marshes or the soil. I concluded that if such convection exists it ought to diminish, like light or gravity, as the square of the distance from the source so that, for instance, "a square yard of (boggy) soil at the distance of one yard will infect as much, *ceteris paribus*, as a square mile of soil at the distance of one mile will." It was a logical critique of these old medical dogmas. Thus in discussing the alleged effects of "climate" on malaria I remark:

"We see fevers of apparently similar nature in every part of India, no matter how diverse the climate. Speaking from my own experience, I have seen the same or similar fevers in the jungles of Burma, full of decaying vegetation and drenched with heavy falls of rain; in the Andaman and Nicobar islands, covered with jungle, it is true, but where one would think the air would be purified by the incessant and strong sea breezes; on the flat coast of Madras with its rice fields and general irrigation; on the tableland of Bangalore with its bare rocks, scanty soil, rock-bound tanks, absence of luxuriant vegetation, cool and equable climate, and red soil; on the similar black soil tableland of Secunderabad with a ground which seems to dry in a few minutes after the heaviest fall of rain; in the desert of Sindh and the Bolán Pass where there is scarcely a single tree to be seen, where the rain seldom or never falls and the air seems to contain not a particle of moisture; and, lastly, at Quetta, 5500 feet above the sea, a flat plain surrounded by barren mountains, scantily supplied with water by an open running stream. What inferences are to be drawn respecting the effect of climate and so on from such an experience? One remains simply in amazement before the facts. How account for the malaria on the paludal hypothesis in the desert of Sindh? How account for it on the effluvium theory amongst the sea breezes of the

Andamans? How explain its prevalence *everywhere* in spite of such difference of climate, soil, vegetation, and moisture?" We can now explain these things. I finished the essay with the words: "In conclusion, I venture to say that we may shortly expect the discovery of certain facts in connection with Laveran's parasite which will reform our views concerning malaria."

Prophetic, but rash! My motto was *Da nobis lucem, Domine*. The essay is full of considerable reading (at the British Museum Library) and how it could have been completed while I was writing two novels at the same time is a mystery to me now!

My work on natural objects found in the blood was not quite worthless either. I invented several beautiful new methods and at one time held that the "blood plates" may quite possibly be spores of certain kinds of leucocyte! But I have never touched this work again.[23]

Before returning to India I invented a small portable microscope, useful for the high powers but capable of being slung round the shoulder like a pair of binoculars. Mr C Baker, of Holborn, brought it out for me and sold many of the instruments.

During our talks Manson and I frequently discussed the possibility of his doing the required researches at his hospital at the Royal Albert Docks near London, and I remember urging (what was really self evident) that if sufficient human cases were not available he could work with birds' malaria and with English midges and gnats—neither of us seemed to know that mosquitoes *are* gnats! I remember also suggesting the use of incubators; but for reasons which I have forgotten he was unwilling, though I urged such researches again (page 31), and he certainly did not do the work.

It has also been said that he "selected" me to verify his theory. Quite untrue. I selected myself and no one else really touched the work till I had done it.

Really the only point of exigence in Manson's hypothesis was the single fact that the process of "exflagellation" (page 14) never occurs until about 10 minutes after the blood is drawn (and kept liquid)—thus suggesting that it is meant to occur in the stomach of some suctorial insect. But even this was not convincing till Sakharoff and I proved that the process was not merely a death struggle (page 76) and all Manson's secondary speculations based upon it turned out wrong. Yet some people write as if his hypothesis itself sufficed to prove the mosquito theory! It was not a mathematical induction like that of Leverrier and Adams regarding Neptune but only a strong biological working hypothesis.

2

First Experiments. Secunderabad, 1895

On 28 March 1895 I embarked at London on the Peninsular and Oriental steamship *Ballarat* for India; and now commenced the four eventful years of severe labour which solved the malaria problem. The details of the work are recorded minutely: (*a*) in my two manuscript volumes of daily laboratory notes; (*b*) in series of frequent letters to my wife and to Dr Manson and in various other letters; and (*c*) in numerous publications. I wish above all, as one motive for this book, to place the reader exactly in my position, even though he be entirely a layman in these matters. He shall (if I can help him to it) look through my microscope, scribble my notes and letters, and post about over India with me! For this purpose the narrative shall consist chiefly of extracts from letters and notes written in the heat of action. If I fail I can only plead my best endeavours; if I succeed he will at least understand something of the passion of investigation!

The ship was a slow one which touched at Gibraltar, Malta, and Brindisi and I commenced at once, as I wrote to my wife, doing microscope work and pricking people's fingers, much to their amusement; and I hoped soon to get hold of cases of fever. On 6 April I wrote to her: "We arrived at Malta at 7 am yesterday and did not leave till 3 pm. I rushed off to the civil hospital at once, and was directed to go to the naval hospital, which is right across the Grand Harbour. I went there and examined the blood of three Malta fever cases. None of them were malaria cases. I found I had gone to the wrong hospital as there was a man called Hughes who had specially studied Malta fever.... Just as it was time to be leaving I saw Hughes, who turns out to be one of the competitors for the Parkes Prize [which I had just won], a very nice and clever man. He gave me a French tract written by him on Malta fever and we are going to write to each other. I left then and was only just in time for the steamer but did some useful work in the little time at my disposal."

This Malta fever (or undulant fever) is a most prolonged and trying kind of fever which haunts parts of the Mediterranean littoral (and other countries) and was shown by (Sir) David Bruce in 1886 to be due to a minute vegetable organism. In 1895 Captain Hughes, of the Army Medical Service, was studying it further in Malta and in 1897 he published an excellent book upon it. At the time of my visit he was glad to have corroboration from me that the malaria parasites were not present in his cases. He was a fine young officer who was killed a few years later in the South African War. Subsequently the commission of which Bruce was the head proved that the fever is spread by means of goats' milk—altogether a great piece of work.

We proceeded and I wrote: "We have had a delicious voyage along the coast of Italy to Brindisi. On our left we have been passing villages, castles, and ruins, and on our right, far away, there have been the high, snow-covered mountains of Greece. Think of that!" This was the first time I had seen Greece. On 8 April, on leaving Brindisi, we had a closer view. "I should like you to have seen the Isles of Greece. We passed right among them. The captain went a little out of the way (?) in order to run between the islands of Cephalonia and Ithaca (where Ulysses and Penelope lived)! We saw the Gulf of Corinth and Sparta [Peloponnesus] with the mountains covered with snow.... I even believe that we saw Mount Parnassus, where Apollo and the Muses lived. I would not have missed the sight for a great deal but hope that we shall yet be able to see it together some day." It was indeed a glorious evening, that of 8 April, as we steamed across the Gulf of Corinth and watched the rays of the setting sun pointing out one by one those sublime summits—which we identified from the captain's charts—the birthplace of Europe, the very sight of which fills one with ambition! We did indeed visit the spot together in 1896; and I saw it again in 1913 and was torpedoed close by in 1917.

I continued in the same letter (10 April): "I have been working steadily with the microscope, dissecting cockroaches (because they have a parasite something like the malaria parasite) and also preparing experiments for my big piece of work. I see clearly now how important the work in connection with the mosquito is.... But then *does* it (the malaria parasite) occur in the mosquito? If I find it by the end of the year I shall certainly try to get three months' privilege leave and come home to show my specimens and to bring you out." On 15 April, in the Red Sea, I wrote: "I have been working away at the microscope and spent yesterday looking for parasites in a small flying fish; I found several very interesting ones. Also I have been reading a lot of medical work in preparation for the mosquito work; but I have failed in finding a single case of malaria on board, which is a nuisance."

At Aden we transhipped into the *Thames* for Bombay, which we reached on Sunday 21 April. I was obliged to waste two days here before proceeding to Secunderabad, to which station my regiment, the 19th Madras Infantry, had been moved from Berhampur, and I spent the time in looking for malaria cases at the civil hospital. On the 23rd I left for Secunderabad, which we reached at midnight, 24–5th, and I lived there in a bungalow *en garçon* with Captain Thomas, the adjutant, and Lieut Hole, both first rate fellows. We had our mess and there was the Secunderabad Club, where we played golf and tennis; but I kept no ponies as I expected to be put upon special malaria work at any time. It was at the height of the hot weather; the ground was a desert and the wind hot and dry. But after paying the usual ceremonial calls I got to work at once in the best of health and spirits. Probably my first letter to Manson has been lost, but progress is reported in those given below.

First it must be explained (for scientific men) that although 15 years had elapsed since the plasmodia had been discovered by Laveran and nearly 10 years since the structure and habits of the different species in the human body had been elucidated by Golgi, the only person who had yet published a paper on them throughout the great Indian Empire was that pioneer Professor H Vandyke Carter, principal of Grant Medical College, Bombay (*Scientific Memoirs of Medical Officers of the Army of India*, 1887), and he had found them only in nine out of 73 cases clinically diagnosed as malaria. Perhaps other workers had really found them (such as Dr Crombie) without investigating them; but there was much doubt on the point owing to the frequency with which artifacts were then being mistaken for them (page 12). It is amazing that the two official investigators specially employed for years by the Government of India had not observed the parasites (page 140). Carter's admirable paper was published before he knew of the illuminating work of Golgi, which had then only just been published, and I was therefore obliged to spend some time in confirming that work for India and also in looking for possible new Indian species of plasmodia. Moreover, in 1895 our modern methods of staining specimens had not been fully developed and

I therefore worked with *fresh* blood and mosquitoes' tissues, and it was lucky that I did so. My principal object was to study the plasmodia not in man but in the mosquito—a thing which had never been yet attempted. Manson's labours on the filariae in mosquitoes were not much help because these are large parasites of quite a different class to the plasmodia and I had to find out most of the technique for myself. There was nothing to guide me as to which exact species of mosquito was concerned in malaria and I had not even been able to obtain any scientific literature on Indian mosquitoes or even on the classification of mosquitoes (Culicidae) in general. It was necessary to investigate everything *de novo*. First I required cases of *Plasmodium falciparum* with numerous sexual forms (Plate I, figs 11–20) (crescent-spheres, spherules, page 22) in their blood; secondly numbers of mosquitoes bred from the larva; and thirdly I had to persuade the mosquitoes to bite the patients.

The letters were written *currente calamo*, generally after a hard day's work and in time to catch the mail. They are here transcribed exactly from the originals, bad grammar and mistakes included; but I have added some elucidations in square brackets and in notes and present my apologies to the reader for my style. Altogether, from April 1895 to February 1899, I wrote 110 letters to Manson containing almost exactly 1000 words each—or about one word to every 10 people killed by malaria in India alone *every year*—perhaps worth the trouble! Apparently the only one of the letters which has been lost was the first, written in April 1894 from Malta or Brindisi. We begin therefore with the second; and I copy it and the three following ones almost entire because I believe that medical readers will like to see them.

SECUNDERABAD, DECCAN,
1 *May* 1895.

DEAR DR MANSON,

I write to report progress and hope you will excuse size of paper. After leaving Malta I examined the blood of all likely cases on board ship (and none were anything but remotely likely) without any result. The day after reaching Bombay I went to the civil hospital and immediately found a woman with tertian from Ahmedabad, with splenitis but not treated with quinine. The parasites were rare, but I found one in the marginal clot in five minutes. There were only about six in the first specimen, crescents and mature spheroids very deeply pigmented. The same evening and the next morning I found the same forms apparently, and in same state, but had not time to work properly as I had to get luggage through the customs. I have been here now less than a week and though I have been very much occupied in calls and business have spent four days and more with the microscope and out of 11 cases have found five due to the parasite. Carter found nine only during some months. The heat is awful and the wind like the blast of an engine furnace. There were only convalescent cases drenched with quinine in my hospital, so I had to drive three miles to the civil hospital in the heat of the day. There were five cases in one ward, in three of which, though they all had had quinine, I found the parasite in 30 seconds (2nd and 3rd fields) each—crescents and large spheroids deeply pigmented. The two cases in which I did not find it were convalescent and were discharged next day. I immediately made a push for the mosquito. By bad luck hardly one was to be found, the air being *fiery* and the three I caught and put into bottles were too frightened or otherwise unwilling to bite; I had no mosquito net.* Up to date I have failed in getting a single mosquito to lay hold, which I think is because I have had to catch them. I am now breeding numbers and have a net ready for use. The three cases were examined carefully the whole day the next day and I found one of the reasons why I could not find the parasites before. Above 90 °F phagocytosis is so quick that all free forms are gobbled up in *twenty minutes*. I used to take my specimens home generally. I found two beautiful forms ready for flagella [Plate I, fig 17] and had logged their position and moved off to study some crescents; on coming back 10 *minutes* after making the specimen they were both inside phagocytes! Next day in my hospital I found two cases of intraglobular parasites with very fine pigment. Malaria was diagnosed in both cases within one minute each. I am sorry that I foolishly packed your chart in the wrong box, now coming by goods train, so that I cannot quote numbers of forms. Four cases in my hospital have hitherto given negative results, but I am at present engaged in looking at the parasite rather than for it. I am delighted and surprised at numbers of cases and ease with which they have been found. My microscope is invaluable. Have you read Crombie's speech in *Indian Medical Gazette* for March? He (and all the doctors in the country) are furious with Mr Hart's speech. He is trying to throw cold water on microscopic diagnosis of malaria and says that he found the

* I used to put the patient lying down on a bed within a bed net and release the mosquitoes at him inside. Whether I devised this method or Manson had used it previously I cannot remember (see page 13).

parasites in only four cases out of 50 in Calcutta in January. My results within a week and before the fever season give 50%. He talks too of half an hour being required, as if that was the average time—so I am keeping careful notes of time taken for each diagnosis. When present, the parasites generally swarm—one or two in three fields about. Today, however, the two cases in my hospital show not a trace of any, but I am off to them again after sundown. Both are fresh cases with very low fever and much headache. Evidently the laws of these sudden appearances and disappearances must be made out if possible. All the cases are beautiful and I am wild with excitement; but these mosquitoes! They *will not bite*. I tried them on myself for experiment, but having been caught they are frightened, I suppose. I expect a crop of new ones in one of my bottles this evening and hope a fever case will show itself to suit. No flagella been seen as yet; but I certainly saw a spent crescent in one specimen. I believe (or rather think) from what Carter says that they are released almost immediately in a high temperature—but we shall see. The finely pigmented bodies seem to belong to quite a different species from the others. I am touting round the country for cases. The doctor in charge of the policemen refused to transfer them to me for experiment and there are difficulties in the way of my experimenting at his hospital. By bad luck I am engaged for tomorrow.

2 May. All my mosquito grubs have been killed owing to my foolishly putting the bottles in the sun. I have consequently started a new lot, but it is vexatious.... Unfortunately the principal medical officer here seems to be putting me on every duty conceivable, but I shall go and look for cases at the civil hospital again tomorrow....

Yours truly,
RONALD ROSS.

The 19th Madras Infantry was then stationed at a cantonment of Secunderabad called Begumpett, situated close to the outflow of the great tank of Secunderabad. The hospital and the hutments of the men and their families were placed not far from the tank, but the officers' mess and quarters were farther away and our bungalow was about a quarter of a mile from the hospital. The hospital was a one storeyed building containing, I think, two wards, besides offices, and it was here that I did most of my important work. Of course this work was carried out in addition to my duties as regimental surgeon and I had to pay all the necessary expenses in connection with it myself. Crescents, spheroids, flagellates, flagellate bodies were the names which I used for denoting the various stages of the sexual forms of *Plasmodium falciparum*, the so-called malignant parasite (Plate I, figs 11–20). The microscope to which I refer was the one recently invented by myself called the "diagnostic microscope" (page 16) and the chart referred to was one recently invented by Manson, who had cut out a large number of coloured drawings of malaria parasites found in various books, especially in the Italian ones, and had stuck these drawings on a single sheet and had then caused printed copies to be made of the whole lot. The different forms were numbered and he proposed that these numbers should be used by observers to record the forms found by them—a very convenient invention. A little before this date Mr Ernest Hart, Secretary of the British Medical Association, had visited India and had criticised the medical services somewhat strongly and, as will be seen by the letter, some of the doctors were rather offended. The layman should know what phagocytes are. They are certain of the so called white cells of the blood—little independent living masses of protoplasm with nuclei which surround and ingest extraneous bodies such as particles, bacteria, or malaria parasites which have effected an entry into the blood—the process of phagocytosis being easy to watch under the microscope in the case of the malaria parasite and being a very interesting phenomenon. Indeed phagocytes have often been considered to be the policemen of the blood—with this difference, that the phagocyte, instead of arresting the culprit, swallows him on the spot; at least he is the scavenger of the blood. Of course when a patient has been taking enough quinine for some days his plasmodia become so much diminished in number that few or none can generally be found in the small drop of blood taken for a single examination, say, one cubic millimetre—that is, one three millionth part of the total amount of blood in an ordinary man.

SECUNDERABAD, 15 *May* 1895.

DEAR DR MANSON,

The fortnight since I wrote to you has been made up partly by disasters and at last by success. I had a bad case requiring constant attendance; the two ague cases in my hospital ceased to show parasites; when, with much difficulty, I had got two cases out of the bazaar all my mosquitoes died again; and next day when I had got a fresh crop of mosquitoes my two cases ran away because I pricked their fingers, in spite of my giving them a rupee a prick! I now saw that it was necessary to get a sepoy case and so spent a day at another regimental hospital. I examined a number of cases in vain (all being soaked with quinine) but at last cast my eye on a case just come in for dysentery: success—two crescents in specimen—case transferred to my hospital. Next day there were a fair number of crescents (11 May) and nothing else—just the sort of case required—but the mosquitoes would not bite. The temperature was between 90 and 100 °F and as dry as a furnace so that the mosquitoes died shortly after being released from the bottle. Nothing I could do persuaded them to bite. The same happened on the 12th, the crescents *swarming*, three or four in a field, the mosquitoes as obstinate as mules and myself nearly frenzied. I watched specimens, however, and saw that at this temperature the crescents show but little change, only a very few becoming spherical. I did not see a single flagellate body though I must have looked at hundreds of parasites on 11th and 12th; and I saw only a few doubtful spent crescents.

Next day (13 May, my birthday) there was better luck. It had rained at night and the morning 6.30 am was cool—I obtained four full mosquitoes. I also found out how to make the insects bite; that is, by wetting the bed and mosquito net with water—this makes them hungry in a moment. The finger blood was swarming with crescents and crescents only. By an accident I did not know that a mosquito had bitten till an hour after he had done so. I bottled him, smoked him (or rather *her*), and separated the abdomen just as you had described; but it was now so hot and dry again and the blood dried almost as soon as squeezed out so that I had to moisten with normal salt solution. Results at once:

1. Parasites present. This was interesting as owing to exceedingly pointed ends of crescents [drawing] I thought they might stick in proboscis.
2. Numbers apparently same as in finger blood (very numerous).
3. Forms, *apparently* nearly all spherules, many spent crescents (?), and very few distinct crescents.

With regard to 3, however, I saw that there were many elements of doubt requiring experiment. I examined the other three mosquitoes within five hours with identical results in all and then set to work to experiment. First, the salt solution which it was necessary to add in all the cases does, I find, turn a large number of crescents into spherules in a minute at this temperature (I believe Laveran says so, but have not time to look him up). In the spherules produced in this manner the pigment granules *swarm* of course for a time; but only once did I observe (in salt solution) a flagellate form and that was unsatisfactory. This showed, however, that the spherules in the mosquito might be due only to the salt solution. Moreover, I noticed that in pure blood, in the marginal clot, the crescents change much more frequently than elsewhere, so I thought that the change in the mosquito might be due to the clotting of the blood (as is likely). As for the *spent* crescents, they seemed very numerous, but I was not certain that they *were* spent crescents. The three forms are [drawings]. In the obscurity of the exuded haemoglobin I could never make out satisfactorily whether the [drawing] spent-looking form had not really a cell wall round it. I noticed no flagellate bodies.

Next day (12th) I spent over six more mosquitoes, much hindered by the rapid drying, trying water, glycerin, Canada balsam, salt solution, etc. In none of the mosquitoes could I get the specimen in the same condition as my control specimens from the finger and I remained unsatisfied both about spherules and spent crescents though I was forced to confess that these *appeared* much *more* numerous and the crescents much *less* numerous than in my control specimens. Today I have been at work on three mosquitoes. One had no parasites, by which I could see that he had got into the net after biting someone else outside (the moisture of the net is attracting outside gentry). The other gave no more certain results, though I got him 20 minutes after biting and examined the blood pure. I have been trying control specimens on ice, too, and found one good flagellate form with *very* delicate flagella, scarcely visible, nothing like the thick flagella I saw with you. I find both spherules and spent crescents in different conditions of the same control specimen, which is irritating because I cannot satisfy myself as to cause. At last this evening, however, my dull brain suggested the proper course—to try dry *smears*. I got a half hour mosquito and smeared his blood with the needle on cover glass, inverted the same after drying in air, and simply laid on slide, using oil-immersion but no medium. *Nothing but spherules*. Not a single crescent and only one or two masses of spent pigment (?). A control finger blood made in same way gave, of course, *all* crescents and no spherules, while a finger blood which had been kept for two hours and was then opened and dried gave *mostly crescents* and a few spherules.

This last experiment then seems to me to *prove* that the crescents undergo change into spherules in the stomach of the mosquito as outside and to *suggest* that they do so faster than in control specimens. I must satisfy myself much more, however, before I state so much definitely. I am, as it were, touching the matter with my soul before my intellect has reached it, just as a phagocyte touches a microbe with its bioplasm while the nucleus lumbers up behind (!). Talk of phagocytosis! I have seen things these last three days but have no time to write about them. I am dead beat now and the lids of my right eye are swollen and painful—at work from 7 am to 7.30 pm with snatches at breakfast and tea.

16 May. Four more hours' work but no good results and have to break off to write mail letters. Certainly crescents are very rare in mosquito's stomach after half an hour, but remain in numbers up to 12 hours in finger blood. Have tried a thick film (to avoid pressure) kept for two hours and then smeared and partly stained [finger blood]. Numbers of crescents, many spherules, and some clusters of pigment. I hope by degrees to improve my manipulation and get a clear certainty whether crescents do or do not transform more quickly in mosquitoes than in specimens.

I mentioned that two men in my hospital had different looking parasites to other cases. These on reference to Marchiafava turn out to be exactly like his tertian, while the others are quartan seemingly; but I must work it out when I have time. I sent your charts to government the other day, with letter asking them to buy for hospitals.

A few days ago I saw Lawrie, who read me part of a letter from Hehir in which he said he found 30% of the corpuscles infected in a case of malaria. One third!... To close, I want to try an experiment—keep an infected mosquito for a week in a bottle containing water and then drink mosquito and water together. But it ought to be tried systematically. I shall get a number of mosquitoes in bottles tomorrow. Case still swarming with crescents—no fever.

Believe me,
Yours truly,
R Ross.

Secunderabad, 22 *May* 1895

Dear Dr Manson,

On the 17th (the day after I finished my last letter) I made another dry smear of mosquito blood which, like the former one, showed spherules and pigment only. On staining it with water solution of methylene blue without fixing, the cellular structure of the spherules was shown more clearly and they looked very different to similarly stained specimens of (*a*) fresh blood and (*b*) blood that had been kept liquid for two hours and then smeared and dried, the former of which gave, as before, only crescents and the latter mostly crescents and a few spherules and pigment masses.

This confirmed me in the view that crescents are transformed much more certainly into spheres in the mosquito's stomach than in specimens. I now determined, however, to make another attempt at liquid specimens because I hate dry smears; so I thought it out and gave the patient instructions to let the mosquitoes fill themselves completely, while I provided myself with a small pair of tweezers with which I could squeeze out the mosquito's stomach with one hand while I held the cover glass with the other, ready to clap on. The result was my first perfect specimen of mosquito blood. About 20 minutes (?) had elapsed since the mosquito had begun sucking and the haemoglobin was of course much diffused. The blood swarmed with perfect spherules, not very large (about 6 μm in diameter) but showing an almost eruptive movement of the pigment as if flagella were about to burst forth in a moment. I looked in vain for flagellated organisms; not one was to be seen, to my surprise. In a very few minutes the pigment oscillation (the intensity of which was much greater than in the control specimens) began to quiet down. Many of the spheres were *shaking*, but, as I have said, not one was flagellate. The general view, however, was very different from an ordinary specimen. All the spheres had *perfect* circular contours and I now noticed that they seemed to be in much larger numbers than in finger blood (contrary to my first impressions). Here are my notes, in thin fields mostly: 7. 3. 9. 7. 2. 2. 3. 2. 2. 0. 2. 2. 1. The fields were consecutive ones and the numbers will give you some idea of the quantity of parasites. I made a specimen of a second mosquito three quarters of an hour after beginning to suck and the results were precisely the same.

On counting the numbers of crescents, spheres, and masses of pigment respectively I obtained:

	Crescents	Spheres	Pigment
1st specimen	7	80	8
2nd specimen	14	30	9
2nd specimen next day after 19 hours	0	8	32 (?)

In both these the number of crescents is a great deal too favourable because it was possible to examine field after field without finding one. Of course the blood last sucked by the mosquito would contain most crescents.

Next day (18th) I began with a finger blood specimen, which gave when fresh:

Crescents and ovals	Spheres	Pigment masses
39	10	1

Then I made two more liquid mosquito specimens at about half an hour, my 18th and 19th mosquitoes.

Up to date I had observed only two flagellate bodies, both in finger blood. I was astonished I did not meet more. Always the spheres seemed ripe for flagella, but they did not come (temperature of air 95 °F). Now, directly I looked at mosquito 18 I saw flagellate organisms in every field. I saw nine altogether in a few minutes, but instead of counting them I wasted my time looking at them. Two fields held two each and I could have found numbers, I do not doubt, if I had looked at once over the specimen. As it was, the spectacle afforded by mosquito 18 was amazing. All the spherules seemed bursting with excitement and exceedingly numerous. In contiguous fields I noted:

$$6.\ 10.\ 8.\ 7.\ 10.\ 14.\ 12.\ 16 = \frac{83}{8} = 10{\cdot}0.$$

But when I came to examine special fields I found 60 parasites in one field and *seventy-two* in the next! All swarming and ready to burst. I think you will confess that no one has had such an experience as this in finger blood. On looking through mosquito 19 I found the same swarms of spheres but no flagellate organisms. I lit a cheroot, went home (though it was only 12 noon), and slept for three hours; the spectacle of flagella had ceased after about 10 minutes.

Next day (19th) I began with mosquito 20 of yesterday. Mostly pigment masses but about 20% still cellular. At 11.50 I made specimen of a fresh mosquito (21) at half an hour with a presentiment of what I was going to see:

4 flagellates in 1st field of 20 spheres
5 ,, in a field of 12 spheres
3 ,, in a field of 10 spheres.

Flagellate organisms everywhere; one or two in every field. I must have seen 30 or 40 though I examined only a few fields, being hardly able to tear myself away from individual organisms. The flagella were excessively fine, quite invisible in open spaces, and seen in haemoglobinous serum and clot; but the flagellate organisms were unmistakable because they were being dragged about all over the field generally or were quivering and being shaken as a dog shakes a rat. The manifestation nearly ceased in a few minutes, though I saw flagellates for half an hour afterwards. Mosquitoes 22 and 23 at 70 and 90 minutes gave no flagellates and but few parasites comparatively. The patient was put under the net again. Mosquito 24 gave results at half an hour as mosquito 21—five flagellates in one field of 12 parasites. Flagellate organisms everywhere, especially in open parts (?). Manifestation lasted in its intensity only for about five minutes.

On 20th and today I did not observe anything new and I did not work yesterday....

23 May. Another disaster among my mosquito grubs owing to the heat I suppose. All dead, but a crop of small mosquitoes which seem *all to be males* and won't bite!

As mail goes today I will close with summary of results. I am inclined on the whole, after examining 28 mosquitoes, to gather that the stomach of the mosquito is very probably the natural locus for the crescent-spherule-flagella metamorphosis [Plate I, figs 13, 15, 17, 19] and I base my opinion on the following five reasons.

1. The number of parasites in mosquitoes appears to be greater than in finger blood (especially in some mosquitoes).* In mosquito 18 I found fields of 60 and 72, as I have said; but in a control of the same time the largest number found in a field was 14. Further study is required.

2. It is certain (and very important) that in mosquitoes at half an hour after beginning to suck practically all the crescents have turned into perfect spheres, whereas in control specimens which have been kept for half an hour and much longer 70% of the parasites remain crescents and ovals (90–100 °F).

3. In the mosquito the pigment of the spheres seems more scattered and much more alive than in finger blood, while almost all the spheres are in this swarming condition when the specimen is first made, whereas in controls many motionless spheres are seen.

4. In the large number of controls [of finger blood] examined carefully by me I have only seen three flagellate organisms (one yesterday) (temp 90–100 °F), whereas out of 11 good mosquito specimens I must have seen 60 or 70 at a modest figure, and these, all but one, in three mosquitoes, 18, 21, 24, and might have seen many more

* Because blood in mosquitoes is more concentrated owing to absorption of the fluid by the insect's digestion.

had I rushed through the specimens quickly enough. On two occasions I saw five flagellates in a field.

5. The phenomenon of exflagellation appears to be going on when the specimen is made and certainly ceases a few minutes afterwards. I have not yet watched a single spherule becoming flagellate, however ripe it has appeared for that development.

I must now cease, Dr Manson, as I have numbers of letters to write; but cease with regret because I could write much more. I propose for the present to go over and over these points as opportunity affords, but alas! the wonder case which fortune has sent me is *drying up* and I may be ordered off to Patiala in a day or two. I may tell you that after seeing mosquito 18, and much more after mosquitoes 21 and 24, I *felt* that practically the first step was assured, but I don't care to be incautious. You can imagine my excitement during the week; yet as I have been able to make step after step I have had a presentiment of what was coming. Of course the principal excitement was over the flagellate organisms. I *knew* that I would get them in 18 and still more in 21. The *first* mosquito of a batch examined will, I think, nearly always yield flagellates, the rest none—why? But the mosquito ought to be killed within half an hour. I leave you to judge as to value of evidence but must state that every point that you predicted seems to come true. Certainly there is nothing contrary to the theory and certainly neither iced nor deep control specimens show anything like the same degree of crescent-sphere-flagella metamorphosis as is seen in the mosquito. I look upon these observations to be as much yours as if you had made them* and if you think they will in any way advance the first steps of the mosquito-malaria theory please make use of them. They are facts but require sifting. Presently I shall give infected mosquitoes, and the water they have died in, to natives on payment and see results; then for seeing where the flagella go to. You will be very pleased with the following. The Maharajah of Patiala in the Punjab (whose medical officer, Surgeon Major Owen, CIE, CMG, I wrote to) has written officially to the government asking for my services from 1 June to 1 November to investigate the fevers which abound in his country! What an opportunity. But government may possibly object: in which case I will ask you to help me in the *BMJ*.† I received a very nasty letter from headquarters which knocked me over on 21st.‡ I have found another typical spring tertian

* They could all have been made in England.

† Manson had informed me that he was adviser for tropical diseases, or something of the kind, to the *British Medical Journal*.

‡ I had applied for civil employment, but not through the "prescribed channel."

in my hospital. I laughed at Hehir for his 30% infected corpuscles but see that Marchiafava notes 50%.

Kind regards to Mrs Manson.

Yours truly,

R Ross.

Are you trying gnats at home? Is any one else working at mosquito? [compare page 16].

SECUNDERABAD, 28 *May* 1895.

DEAR DR MANSON,

I think that my last letter missed the post owing to the date of sailing having been advanced one day without sufficient notice; I am not sorry, because my former observations were somewhat erratic and I have now been able to put in five days of more methodical and satisfying work. I have been going over and over the same ground and have been able, I think, to reach some definite conclusions respecting the first step of the metamorphosis inside the mosquito.

After writing I determined to follow your advice exactly, get a batch of full mosquitoes, and examine one after the other at short intervals. On the 24th I obtained a batch of six mosquitoes all of which had begun biting nearly at the same moment—that is, directly the patient was put into the net. They were now dissected and examined with the utmost rapidity possible at intervals of 8, 22, 40, 60, 120, and 180 minutes after they had begun to bite. The results were: [details of mosquitoes 29 to 34.]

The above is taken from notes made between each mosquito. Before beginning the process I made a sealed control specimen from the finger which, together with mosquitoes 29–32, I re-examined whenever I had time in order to watch and compare progress *pari passu*.

25 May. The process repeated. [Details of mosquitoes 35 to 40.]

The above, with all my former experiments, had now given me a very good idea of what occurs in mosquito's stomach. Sunday 26th I set aside for experiments with haemocytometer—of which later. On 27th and 28th (today) the whole course of the 24th and 25th was repeated to make absolutely sure.

The result is that I can now make a definite statement of the life history of the parasite from its being drawn in to some hours later; and this with the greater certainty because the experiments invariably confirm each other with but trifling differences.

... The progress of things, then, is this.

1. Almost all the crescents are converted into spheres very shortly after they enter the mosquito's stomach. Sometimes a fair number may be found at 10, 15, 20 minutes or even more; but these are almost always *seen in the same part of the specimen* and therefore belong probably to the *last intake of blood*. It is very rare to find more than *one* or *two* crescents in a whole specimen made at a longer interval. Ovals are not often seen. Untransformed crescents are, I believe, injured or aborted ones.

2. The spheres are always found. They have a perfect contour and contain a clear fluid which distinguishes them markedly from the masses of corpuscles in the midst of which they are generally found. At first their pigment is clustered together; then the outermost pigment particles begin to oscillate; lastly all the pigment particles commence swarming, while the whole cell may take on a slight jerking rotatory movement.

3. Flagellate organisms may be found from 7 to 38 minutes or more. When seen they lie almost always in great numbers in *contiguous fields*, suggesting that they belong to the *same intake* of blood and have *ripened* at the same time. They are always, so far as I have experienced, found within a minute or two of the lens being brought to a focus (my first survey being very rapid). The whole manifestation ceases in a very few minutes. Owing to this last fact, and possibly owing to the *process of making the specimen allowing the flagella to free themselves*, they are sometimes not to be found (?).

4. The spent pigment masses* may sometimes be seen very early, even at 8 minutes, but then are *very few* in number. This number steadily increases, almost without fail, in successive mosquitoes until, as in mosquito 39, they may reach 65% of all the parasites (not enclosed in phagocytes). Their appearance is quite characteristic, simply because they are not enclosed in the clear cells of the spheres. They are easily seen to be mere dead clusters of pigment (sometimes with very feeble oscillations). They may be masses, rings, or *drawn out* clusters. Their absence in the earliest mosquitoes and their large numbers in the latest show conclusively that they are due to a progressive metamorphosis inside the mosquito and not to *crushing* in making the specimen, but many of them may be pigment *rejected* by phagocytes which have swallowed spheres; I think Mannaberg allows this.

5. Phagocytes containing spheres and pigment begin to be seen later than the spent pigment, at about 20 minutes or so, and increase in number up to about two hours.

* That is, the crescent-sphere (Plate I, fig 19) *after* the flagella have escaped from it, leaving only a number of pigment granules within a collapsed little bag.

6. About 30 or 40 % of the parasites *fail* in *throwing out flagella* and remain as spheres,* the pigmentary movements gradually becoming slower and slower, the pigment collecting in a heap to one side and then (two hours) the bioplasm beginning to swell up irregularly (Laveran's old corps, No 3).

The above developments may be shortly stated in two sentences—

(A) Practically *all* the crescents become spheres a few minutes after being taken into the mosquito's stomach.

(B) From 30 to 40 % of the spheres *die* after one or two hours, the rest having either given out flagella, been eaten by phagocytes, or simply broken up (?).

29 May. These observations, then, prove conclusively that the crescent-sphere-flagella metamorphosis *does* go on inside the mosquito, which I think you said was to be considered as the first step in the theory. But it may now be said with reason that this does not prove that the stomach of the mosquito is the *natural locus* of the metamorphosis because a similar metamorphosis may be seen to occur whenever the blood is drawn from the patient and allowed to remain still for a sufficient period. Against this objection I will state that the *metamorphosis proceeds to a much greater degree in the mosquito than in control specimens of finger blood.*

Firstly, the number of crescents which, in a finger blood specimen, become spheres varies much in different specimens made at the same time and also in different parts of the same specimen. I think you will agree with me that from 10 to 70 % of the parasites remain crescents. Thus this morning I made two good controls, in the first of which the crescents were only about 10 % after 35 minutes, while in the second, made shortly afterwards, the crescents numbered from 60 to 70 % after half an hour. In short it seems that the crescent-sphere metamorphosis is greatly influenced by certain local conditions of the specimen;† but it may be stated confidently that a very fair number of undeveloped crescents are always to be found in finger blood even after the lapse of many hours. This is not the case in the mosquito; here practically *no crescents* are to be found after half an hour or so. In fact I am prepared to state that I can distinguish at sight between a specimen which has been made directly from the finger and one in which the blood has passed for six or 10 minutes through the mosquito's stomach.

* These are now known to be the *females*. I thought that they were parasites which had died without throwing out "flagella" (sperms).

† See page 77 for the reasons.

Secondly, I have remarked already on the greater violence of pigmentary movements in the mosquito.

Thirdly, since my last letter I have found flagellates in control specimens much more readily because I now know exactly the period when to look for them (10 to 20 minutes). Still I have never seen anything like the numbers witnessed in mosquitoes 18, 21, 24, 44, 46.

Fourthly, a curious proof from the effect of *quinine*. Patient had 15 gr on 27th and 10 gr yesterday morning. In my preliminary control of yesterday I was astonished to find hardly any of the crescents transformed and, since I had seen the same before after quinine, I thought that all the crescents had been killed. On examining my first mosquito at 10 minutes I again found all the parasites *crescents*. This was quite contrary to all former observations and I was now getting certain that the crescents were indeed dead until, on examining my next mosquito at 20 minutes, I observed that the proportion of spheres was much greater, though crescents were still much commoner than they ought to have been. Successive mosquitoes gave fewer and fewer crescents until after 69 minutes there were only three in the whole specimen, while the sphere-pigment metamorphosis had gone on as before. Returning now to my original control I found all the crescents still there and no pigment masses. From which I conclude: quinine *checks completely* the crescent-sphere evolution in finger blood but only *delays* it in the mosquito. In other words the mosquito's stomach has the power, apparently, of resuscitating parasites paralysed by quinine. Of course the effect of quinine on flagellate organisms has long been given, but it is generally stated that it has no effect on crescents.*

On Sunday 26th I made some laborious attempts to estimate number of parasites in mosquito blood with haemocytometer. These all failed owing to difficulty of obtaining *enough* blood and dryness of air. I estimated parasites in finger blood at 1 to 410·3 corpuscles—that is, 8000 parasites and 3 282 400 corpuscles in a cubic millimetre of blood (my first attempt was computed wrongly). Number of parasites still appears to me to be generally much greater in mosquito, but I cannot get proof.†

I have only seen one free flagellum but some curious things. Do you think it possible that all the flagella are coils of a single long animal inside the sphere (?). Hardly possible. Tomorrow I begin second step—watching the flagella. Please send me advice. I watched a sphere this morning break up and become spent pigment apparently without

* I became less positive on these points later.

† See footnote, letter of 22 May 1895, page 31.

exit of flagellum. Parasites continue decreasing slightly in numbers. Have dissected 54 mosquitoes up to date. My Parkes Gold Medal arrived. No further news from Patiala. Three more cases of tertian parasite in my hospital. On 25th I made a certain experiment on two men of which you may hear later. Every one of your predictions has come true.

With kind regards,

Yours truly,

R Ross.

3
False Scents. Secunderabad, 1895

Thus within one month I had been able to show that the crescent-sphere-flagella phenomenon occurs in the mosquito's stomach not only just as it does in blood from the finger, but much more frequently and simultaneously—suggesting that the mosquito's stomach is the natural *locus* for this surprising metamorphosis.

During my stay in India Manson wrote me 55 letters, from 17 May 1895 to 18 January 1899, exactly half the number I wrote to him. I should like to print all of them but do not feel justified in giving more than a few extracts directly concerned with my work. Here are some from his first two replies.

21 Queen Anne Street
Cavendish Square,
17 *May* 1895

My Dear Ross,

I was delighted to get your letters from Malta and from Secunderabad and to gather from them that you pursue the plasmodium with enthusiasm. You do not lack for material and energy, and though you may get many a check I firmly believe you will work out some important result; you cannot fail to do so. Let this conviction fill your mind when inclined to despond, and look on a stone wall as a stimulant rather than as an insuperable barrier to progress. I have run my head against them often enough, but somehow if I kept hammering at it and thinking about it, sooner or later I got over or under or through when I had set my mind to it; and so will you....

Already you have proved that Crombie is wrong and that a diagnosis of malaria can be made with the microscope in less than five minutes. You must set them right about this in the first place....

Soon I expect to hear that you have followed the plasmodium into the mosquito or some other suctorial insect. If you succeed in this you will go up like a shot and get any facilities you may ask for in the way of leisure for investigation and laboratory appliances and assistance. I only wish I were you.

I am full up with preparing lectures for my course on tropical diseases at St George's. I hate the labour of writing, but I am in for it and have got to get it done somehow. My first lecture is next Tuesday. I have promised 20—two a week—but so far have only some eight or nine ready. I wish they were all written.

In consequence of this work and a good deal to do in the way of practice I have not had much chance for further work at malaria. Indeed patients have been few for the last two months. I got a guinea-worm case some time ago and have on hand a rare lot of infected cyclops.* It is really a very pretty experiment. I had some photo-micrographs made of the cyclops by Pringle. They show the embryos in the interior of the cyclops very well indeed. I shall try to get a spare one to send you one of these days....

Bakers are going to lend me six of your microscopes for my lectures. They will be well advertised therefore and I shall show my gratitude to you and to Baker by giving them a puff. He has already sold a considerable number and is now making a dozen [page 16].

Hoping to hear again from you soon and assuring you of my sympathies in your work and willingness to help you in any way I can,

I remain,
Yours very truly,
PATRICK MANSON.

21 QUEEN ANNE STREET,
CAVENDISH SQUARE,
21 *June* 1895.

MY DEAR ROSS,

I am exceedingly obliged for your letters. I look forward to receiving them with the greatest interest and when a mail passed without getting one the other day I was terribly disappointed for I thought you had fallen

* Fedschenko's cycle, see page 13.

sick or that you had got a check or that you had given up the quest. Above everything don't give it up. Look on it as a Holy Grail and yourself as Sir Galahad and never give up the search, for be assured you are on the right track. The malaria germ does not go into the mosquito for nothing, for fun, or for the confusion of the pathologist. It has no notion of a practical joke. It is there for a purpose and that purpose, depend upon it, is its own interests—germs are selfish brutes.

Your finds are most interesting and encouraging. The mere fact that the parasite is not digested is enough to prove to my mind that it is in its proper habitat, and the fact you have discovered that it advances in development more rapidly and more frequently in the mosquito's stomach is confirmatory of this inference. But now the struggle to advance the next step begins. What next to look for and where to look.

I think you would do well to prepare a series of stained preparations from mosquito blood illustrative of what you have already done. I think that such a series of preparations would show the progress of development better than anything else as they could be made so rapidly at a few minutes' interval and could then be stained and examined at leisure. If you have time do this and if you are generously inclined send me a series either in bottle or stained or both....

About the next step. Among other things examine the dung the little yellow specks you see on the glass the insect is kept in for evidence of malarial products. It may contain nothing, but it is easily examined. Then I should examine the ova of the mosquito from time to time before and after they are deposited in the water, for I have an idea that the beast gets into them and so into the larva and becomes more or less a permanent parasite not only in the individual mosquito that sucked him in but in the progeny of this mosquito. This will be a more difficult matter. Then I should keep mosquitoes to maturity and tease them up in salt solution and examine their tissues one by one, searching inside all cells for something like the plasmodium. I question if he will be pigmented, but I am fairly sure that he is intracellular. This too will be a long and difficult task. But it is not without hope. Look about the kidney tube or the analogous structure among the long caecal tubes, about the little corpuscles representing the blood corpuscles in the walls of the stomach and in the muscles of the thorax. Compare malaria-fed mosquitoes with non-malaria-fed mosquitoes and compare their progeny.

If you would experiment, create an artificial marsh by allowing the water in which the mosquito has died and laid her eggs and in which her progeny have been swimming about to dry up, then pulverise this and get someone to inhale the dust you stir up from it. Or drink it suspended in water. The experiments would be interesting but perhaps not altogether safe. *Dulce et decorum est pro patria mori.* But don't do it yourself.

My guinea-worms are still alive in the cyclops and slowly undergoing changes. It is now over six weeks since they entered the crustacean and they are still quite lively, only casting their skins and dropping their tails according to last report three days ago. I hope you will have a chance of a fling at this subject as well as at malaria and filaria.

I must close my letter now as I have a lot to do this afternoon and don't want to miss the post or to let you suppose that I don't take a great interest in your work and to give you an excuse of not writing to me.

With all good wishes for continued success,

Yours very sincerely,

PATRICK MANSON.

This last letter reached me before 10 July, by which time, as will be seen, I had already begun to try to infect human beings by water from an "artificial marsh" and to search the tissues of mosquitoes for parasites similar to the plasmodium—it was too early as yet to search their eggs and evacuations. Of course all these suggestions were obvious to anyone who was thinking seriously of the subject, and Manson seems to have forgotten that we had already talked them over in England.

Thus far Manson's induction had carried me triumphantly along, but it already began to fail me as a clue. He had supposed that the so-called flagella (Plate I, fig 21) are flagellated spores—that is, actively motile bodies which could work their way through the stomach wall of the insect in order to live in the tissues where, he thought, they grow in some unknown position into an unknown form. Still later, he surmised, they escape from the insect into the water when she dies on that fluid and thence infect any person who happens to drink it. But if all this had been true I should now have been able to observe large numbers of the alleged flagellated spores wriggling about everywhere in the contents of the stomach. I was much disappointed at not finding them, though I did not like to disappoint Dr Manson equally by telling him so at this early stage of the investigations (but see letter of 10 July). I still hoped that something curious happened to the flagella which enabled them to escape my oil-immersion lens. That indeed was the case; they are not flagellated spores at all but sperms (Plate I, fig 22)—but this was not found out for two years more.

In the meantime, however, I had thought of a short cut. If Manson's hypotheses were sound (and the mosquitoes were of the proper species) water in which a mosquito which had bitten a case of malaria happened to die should infect healthy persons after a few days; and I had already tried the experiment—as will now appear. It is an example of the tricks which fortune plays upon investigators that my first experiment appeared successful. But it was a mere accident—many subsequent cases failed entirely to react.

The mosquitoes with which I was working were either my *grey* or *brindled* mosquitoes (see page 99)—that is, genus Culex or Stegomyia. As I have said, I could obtain no literature on mosquitoes at all at that time even when I was in England except a non-zoological article in an encyclopaedia. The large majority of the insects used in the above experiments were stegomyia.

A paper by me describing all this work[24] was subsequently read before the South Indian Branch of the British Medical Assocation in December 1895 and was published also in the *Indian Lancet* in 1896. Neither of these publications is easily accessible in Britain or abroad.

SECUNDERABAD, 5 *June* 1895.

DEAR DR MANSON,

I am in a state of great excitement and have no time to write you a full letter this week as the post goes out today. One of my "certain experiments" which I mentioned has come off.

On 17 May I took four full mosquitoes from the crescent case, Abdul Kadir, and put two in one bottle and two in another with a little water. They were kept in a cool place until 25 June [May], when they were found dead on the surface of the water. In one of the bottles very small mosquito grubs were found, showing that the mosquitoes' eggs had been hatched. The contents of this bottle, minus the dead bodies of the mosquitoes, was given to a native, Lutchman, on 25 May at 8 pm on payment, after full explanation of the nature of the experiment. The contents of the other bottle was given to another native in a similar way. I think myself justified in making this experiment because of the vast importance a positive result would have and because I have a specific in quinine always at hand.

Lutchman is 20 years old, a healthy looking young fellow who *says* that he has never had fever. Yesterday he was all right. This morning at 8 am (exactly 11 days from drinking the water) he came to the hospital assistant complaining of headache. Temp. 99·8° F. Looking ill.

Temperature has been taken every half hour and rose to 101·4° F at noon, since when (1.30) it has been declining. This looks very promising. Incubation agreed closely with former experiments. The type ought to be either quotidian or summer tertian according to Marchiafava etc (crescents), which do not necessarily begin with rigor. Headache considerable. Three specimens carefully examined give no results, but such are not yet to be expected. If temperature rises again this afternoon it may be summer tertian. Chances are greatly against accidental fever because out of the whole regiment I am getting only three or four cases weekly; these are always either spring tertians or *no parasite* (not carefully examined). Anyway, if the attack is quite ephemeral the result will be interesting. A third man drank mosquito water on 31 May....

Yours truly,

R Ross.

The letter concludes with some work confirmatory of previous results and a postscript on Lutchman's temperature on 5 June, taken half-hourly up to 2.30 pm.

SECUNDERABAD, 10 *June* 1895.

DEAR DR MANSON,

Many thanks for your letter of 17 May—but first about the man Lutchman. He had three days' fever, but I failed entirely in finding any parasites in his blood. His temperatures were....

[Here follows a table of hourly temperatures from 8 am to midnight, taken on 5, 6, 7 June. The highest temperature reached was 103·0 ° F at 5 pm on the 5th and 100° F on the 6th, after which it fell to normal except for a very slight rise on the 7th.]

This gives three rises—at 8 am on 5th, at 3 pm on 6th and at 11 am on 7th. The first attack lasted 20 hours. Clearly it was intermittent fever possibly of a mild postponing summer tertian type. There was headache but neither rigor nor splenic tenderness. Bowels constipated first day. No medicines given. Repeated examinations of the best possible fields of flattened smooth round corpuscles failed to show any parasites at all....

12 June. No parasites in Lutchman's blood and no more fever. Neither of the other men has had fever. I am at present, as ill luck has it, getting no cases of parasites and so have been dissecting a mosquito or two, pricking fingers at random, and playing golf. The rains have broken and

it is only 88° F in the verandah at noon. I found a beautiful double tertian some miles from here but the man was too ill to be moved. The doctor asked me to look at the blood as he thought it was a *funny case*....

In several mosquitoes I find bodies like this drawing [see figure on page 52] which seem to me to be parasites, perhaps coccidia. They are about 20 μm in length and were very numerous....

Do you think that you would like to come out to Patiala instead of to Demerara [page 45]? I should like to sound Owen about it if I go there....

In specimens made after your method [Laveran's method] we get five different kinds of field which I find it very useful to distinguish thus:—

Field A. Very thin. The haemoglobin is crushed out of the corpuscles and forms a thin homogeneous yellow fluid containing only shadows of corpuscles.

Field B. A little deeper. All the corpuscles are smooth, not crushed nor vacuolated, lying separate or tessellated; the serum is clear. This is the best field for intracorpuscular forms.

Field C. The corpuscles lie fairly separate but are crushed and vacuolated owing to no pressure being exerted on them by the cover glass.

Field D. The corpuscles are in rouleaux. Good for crescents and crescent-sphere-flagella metamorphosis.

Field E. The marginal clot of drying blood. Good for all sorts of pigment masses.

Have you ever seen a phagocyte take in a whole swarming sphere and burst it as we burst grapes between the tongue and palate? I have, several times. It is done in an instant. Another point—the quinine and fever forms described by Mannaberg occur, I think, only after the specimen has been made for some 20 minutes.

With kind regards, believe me,

Yours truly,

R Ross.

I shall write you again when I have *something to say*.

The parts of this letter not printed give a tabular summary of my results with the man Abdul Kadir which were described in previous letters. The parasites in his blood now began to diminish rapidly and I was forced to search elsewhere for cases.

SECUNDERABAD, 5 *June* 1895.

DEAR DR MANSON,

...I brought back Abdul Kadir to my hospital since he still has a few crescents, but I was allowed to have him for only two days. I went through the "course" twice, however. It appears useless to repeat this process on the man (I have done it eight times now) because the results are invariable in every experiment. The man has been having much quinine lately and consequently the crescents scarcely transform at all in finger blood specimens. They remain unchanged for an hour or more (temperature of air 75° F) and then perhaps one out of four or five becomes a sphere. I saw one flagellated body with eight distinct flagella. What now is so remarkable is that in the mosquitoes they are *all* transformed in 20 minutes at most. In six mosquitoes containing about 15 to 20 parasites each I found only *one* crescent—all the rest were spheres or spent pigment. In these cases I examined the mosquitoes as well as the controls most thoroughly and deliberately and I am absolutely *certain* now of the great effect produced by the insect's stomach on the crescent-sphere transformation, at least so far as I can judge by one case alone (Abdul Kadir). It is a remarkable and significant fact.

There is much to be studied in the exflagellation process (shall we call it ecdysis?). In the prisoner I watched a sphere throw out flagella which almost immediately curled up round the cell and stopped moving (certainly within 120 seconds). Mannaberg describes this somewhere. The extreme brevity of the stage in this case shows why one so often misses flagellated organisms. I saw none in my last mosquitoes, though spent pigment masses abounded and showed that the process was occurring. When they *are* found I think they are generally found in *clear* serum. This suggests that in viscid blood the flagella are able to leave the cell so rapidly and easily that scarcely a movement is seen—what do you think? I remember that in mosquitoes 18, 21, and 24 nearly all the flagellate bodies were in pretty clear serum. But why do the flagella sometimes curl up so quickly? Also why do the cells sometimes break up without any flagella at all? Have you seen this? Why have I seen so few free flagella in the mosquitoes?*...

... in May and June I have found altogether six spring tertians, two quartans, three summer tertians, five crescent cases, and one with an undetermined fever form—17 cases. What has made me rather conceited is that most of my 20 negative cases mentioned in postcard turned out

* Because many of them were entering the female spheres at once.

to have a curious *continued* fever lasting four or five days. They all began in a batch after the first heavy rains. On the whole I don't think I can have actually missed the parasite in more than four or five true malaria cases—and this though I made no persistent search. In fact I am inclining to the view that when the parasites are present they can usually be found in two or three minutes at most....

Have got six mosquitoes from Abdul Kadir maturing in order to give to a man. About 15 or 20 parasites in each. I shall give them all together. No crescent in Lutchman, nor any more fever.

Yours truly,
R Ross.

SECUNDERABAD, 10 *July* 1896.

DEAR DR MANSON,

During the last fortnight I have not been able to find a single fresh case of malaria, though I have been hunting all round the station for them.... I have looked in all sorts of cases for crescents without result. In spite of offering rewards to hospital assistants of the civil and other hospitals I can't get a case. I thought I should find cases in the civil hospital the other day to a certainty but was disappointed. I don't know what's up with the place. Yet there are tanks and marshes everywhere and only a scanty rainfall. The huts of my regiment are practically just over a great tank with muddy, drying margin—yet out of 800-odd men, no malaria. I will tell you why—because the mosquitoes don't thrive this windy weather. I will bet on your suggestion that malaria is in the first place a disease of mosquitoes—hence the idea of it being carried by winds. It is the *mosquito* and not the *germs* which are carried by the wind. They probably deposit the germs in the drinking water. This is the reason why I am beginning to work with drinking water instead of with an artificial marsh as you suggest. If the germs were so numerous in the air as to infect one person they ought to infect *many*; this will not explain isolated cases satisfactorily. It appears much more likely that only those persons are infected who have drunk water by chance out of a chatty or water pot in which an infected mosquito has laid her eggs—the infected mosquito may of course have been blown from a marsh, where the disease is rife among the mosquitoes, or may have recently bitten a malaria case. During windy weather mosquitoes don't thrive....

Why did not I find more *free* flagella? Either they dash away into the tissues at once or, I am beginning to think, cease to move almost as soon as they free themselves from the cysts (footnote, page 43). They have to scurry out of the cyst for fear of the phagocytes but after that may develop without movement in the contents of the stomach—again what do you think? Oh for another case! I make this conjecture because there ought to be numbers of free active flagella in mosquito's blood, whereas I saw only two or three, while on the other hand they may be seen to cease moving in a few minutes. In mosquitoes 18, 21, and 24 there ought to have been swarms of free flagella apparent *if they had continued wriggling*. I think that this point requires study before attacking the question of the tissues; I shall work with much thinner films than, for fear of bursting the spheres, I did before. Don't you think that the flagella ought first to be found free in the stomach? Staining etc must be tried. As soon as this is done I shall go on to follow your advice exactly about the tissues....

Tomorrow morning I am going to see some horses said to have intermittent fever. Am thinking of sending an account of the mosquitoes to the South Indian Branch of the British Medical Association in order to work them up a little. Nobody is doing anything in the microscope line. The Patiala investigation has collapsed entirely owing to opposition of Lieut Governor of Punjab....

With kind regards,

I remain,

Yours truly,

R Ross.

The Patiala business was as follows: Surgeon Major Charles William Owen, IMS, CIE, was Chief Medical Officer to the Maharaja of Patiala, the head of the Sikh nation in Northern India, and was interested in malaria and had corresponded with me before I left for India. On or before the time I reached Secunderabad I had suggested to him that the maharaja might confer a benefit on medical science if he were to apply for my services for the purposes of a special malaria survey in his territory. Of course such a thing at that time had hardly ever been done, but Surgeon Major Owen, with great enterprise, persuaded the maharaja to approve the scheme, and I was expecting to be sent north any day when there came the further news that the Lieutenant Governor of the Punjab had vetoed the proposal on the ground of expense. That ended the matter. In fact I was so favourably placed at Secunderabad for malaria work that I would not have gained much by going north, except money, regimental pay being very small, but I did not know this at first.

The reference to Demerara in my letter of 10 June may also be explained. When I was in England Dr Manson told me that he was proposing to go there for the purpose of working at his mosquito theory himself if only he could have his expenses paid by the Royal Society or some other body that grants funds for such purposes; and I now suggested that perhaps Patiala would take him instead of myself. In his letter of 10 July, however, he told me that the Royal Society declined to give him the grant asked for. All the same I always wondered why he did not make the required studies himself at the Branch Seamen's Hospital at the Royal Albert Dock, of which he was a physician. There were plenty of malaria cases there and malaria mosquitoes (anophelines) abound in the neighbourhood; and indeed I suggested this again in the postscript to my letter of 22 May. As a matter of fact he could easily have done in London all the work that I had been doing in Secunderabad—incubators, mosquitoes, and suitable cases all being available. He had, I think, hoped to prove the theory in a few months' work at Demerara but, as will be seen, he would have found the job a much tougher one than he had expected. The British Medical Association had actually granted him £150 on 16 January 1895 for the proposed visit (see *British Medical Journal* 29 April 1922, p 698).

That Manson himself was thinking of working at his mosquito theory in London is apparent from the concluding extract from the following letter (his third one):

28 *June* 1895.

MY DEAR ROSS,

... My idea about the beast in the mosquito is, as I think I told you, that it is transmitted in a sort of hereditary way from mother mosquito to sons and daughters as a cell parasite, and that it gets to man in mosquito dust—the debris of dead mosquitoes in which the germ has become encysted, that these germs on entering the human mouth or air passages or swallowed in the saliva or what not, or as in your experiment in water, penetrate the human mucous membrane as they do the mosquito's stomach, and so get into his circulation. An experiment I should like to see tried would be to evaporate some water in which malariated mosquitoes had died—say in some small glass bottles; to evaporate it thoroughly so that the sediment will not decompose, but to evaporate it in the sun so as not to scorch it and also so as to resemble what occurs in nature; to have this transmitted to England; to add there a little water to the dried sediment; and then to drink it. I am willing to try. A positive result to such an experiment would be irrefutable. Another experiment worth trying would be to pulverise this same sediment or the bodies of desiccated malariated mosquitoes and then inhale the dust.

A suggestion I would make about these experiments is that the mosquito water or mosquito dust should be taken or inhaled first thing in the morning and on an empty stomach so that there would be no danger of it having its included germs destroyed by the stomach juices.

Pay some attention to the mosquito grubs in malariated mosquito water; it may be that they take in the germ in the water they swallow.

Another hint I would give you. Send specimens of the mosquito for identification of species. Possibly different species of mosquito modify the malaria germ; that the differing degrees of virulence depend on the difference of species of mosquito that has served as alternative host to the parasite....

Simplicity is the best guarantee of success. As little machinery as you can get along with. Let the other fellows, the men who are going to come after you, worry with these things and elaborate in detail the big principles which you indicate and establish. Go for principles—not details too much.

I have not had a malaria case for a month. I hear of some mosquitoes at the docks and if I got my case I should have a try for the malariation of the insect and the consumption of his infusion myself....

I remain,

Yours very truly,

PATRICK MANSON.

SECUNDERABAD, 17 *July* 1895.

DEAR DR MANSON,

Your very pleasant letter of 28 June reached me only yesterday. It is very encouraging to me to get your letters, but you *must not* feel called upon to waste your time in replying to mine unless you have absolutely nothing better to do ... remember that I am an exile with no one to talk to about malaria germs! But you must not waste your time over replying unless you think it necessary....

I am nearly wild and have been able to do nothing for nearly six weeks now. I have been all round the hospitals again and have touts out everywhere and, with great difficulty, have obtained three bazaar people—no crescents. The bazaar people won't come to me though I offer what is enormous payment to them. I offer 2 and 3 rupees for a single finger prick and much more if I find crescents—they think it is witchcraft.... Also, do you know, I believe that I have come upon a new variety altogether but have not observed it sufficiently yet to let you know about it; the corpuscles seemed to be infected with one, two, or three very minute forms.... Perhaps after all they are some kind of vacuole—but they move and turn round!—we will see. [What I called "eye forms" later. Of no consequence (page 71).]

I also examined five horses with fever—chart not intermittent—no parasites seen.

The fourth *experimental case* has had no result (now 15 days). But the malarialised mosquitoes contained only a few parasites each and were kept too long dead I think. Thus only one out of four cases contracted fever and though that fever *looked* like a malarial one (summer tertian—not clear), I could find no parasite. Yet the incubation period was quite correct and when we come to think of all the chances of failure in such experiments we must by *no means* expect success in more than a small percentage of cases, at least at first.... Don't for heaven's sake mention at the British Medical Association that Lutchman is a dhooley-bearer—did I tell you so? He is a government servant. To give a government servant fever would be a crime! (Also, I will add here, to give a lecturer on tropical diseases at two London hospitals guinea-worm would be a worse one.)

You must not think of trying the cyclops. What I suggest is this. Bribe the man at the bar at the House of Commons to put the cyclopses in the drinks of the MPs. It will draw attention to science, put a stop to much useless talking by keeping the MPs off their legs, and not injure anyone of consequence.

With kind regards,

Yours truly,

R Ross.

SECUNDERABAD, 18 *July* 1985.

DEAR DR MANSON,

At last!

Just as I said in my letter yesterday, Abdul Wahab, the man with ring forms and pigmented leucocytes only, showed crescents this morning—one in four fields. At work again. Eight hours today.

I said I was going to watch free flagella [Plate I, fig 21]. With my usual luck I found a beauty in my very first specimen and watched it for three solid hours exactly, without taking my eye off him. So much for my absurd theory of the flagella becoming quiescent. What he did you will think interesting.

He riggled [*sic*] around for 20 minutes like a trypanosome so that I could hardly follow him. Then he brought up against a phagocyte and remained so long that I thought the phagocyte had got hold of him. Not a bit; he was not killed or sucked in but kept poking him in the ribs in different parts of the body. I was astonished; and so, apparently, was the phagocyte. He kept at this for about a quarter of an hour and then went away across two fields and went straight at another phagocyte! He pushed into this in several places with one end for a long time and the phagocyte seemed to rear up and try to get round him but could not. At last the phagocyte seemed to give up and flattened itself against an air bubble, the flagellum still poking away at him. After 50 minutes the beast seemed to be getting tired, when a very curious thing happened; a third phagocyte came at him with mouth open right and straight across the field but had no sooner got near him when the flagellum left his fallen foe and attacked the new one, holding on and shaking like a snake on a dog. In one minute the third phagocyte turned sharp round and ran off howling!!!—I assure you. I won't swear I heard him howling, but I *saw* him howling. He went right across a whole field, the flagellum holding on to his tail like this [drawing]. This continued for five minutes, the poor phagocyte literally *legging it*, after which the flagellum left him and went away. By this time the beast had become more visible and had a large swelling in the middle [drawing]. I watched him steadily and his movements gradually became slower. He was certainly able to attach himself to the cover glass (as shown by touching it with a pen) by *either* end and even perhaps by the swelling. At last this swelling moved to one end [drawing] nearly of the beast and became very large and distinct, until after three hours the creature evidently died—at any rate, curled up and ceased to move. Isn't this interesting? I think it shows first that the phagocytes have no more power over free flagella than over trypanosomes; secondly, the beast was evidently attacking the phagocytes, probably *mistaking them for some other kind of cell**—so I judge by its leaving the phagocytes after a time.

After this I put the mosquitoes on. Results of Abdul Kadir completely

* Absolutely correct. I think it mistook the leucocytes for female plasmodia. Detailed notes and drawings of all these observations are entered in my laboratory diary.

confirmed—and more. The first mosquito was killed at 20 minutes. My usual luck again—*all the parasites were flagellate and there were scores of free flagella.* I say *all* the parasites—all except about 5 % which were spheres. In the second mosquito at 40 minutes I saw four flagellates; the rest were spheres and spent pigment. In neither mosquito was there a single crescent, though in the first control specimen 50 % of the parasites remained crescents after three hours. I killed no more mosquitoes, being tired out, but kept eight for malarialising experiments. After this it is not much use bothering about going over the "first step" again—but I shall make you some sets of specimens and try to stain the flagella; Mannaberg does it. The spectacle of the first mosquito was really wonderful. I shall dream of it. Goodnight. So was the fight between the flagellum and the three phagocytes, I shall write a novel on it in the style of *The Three Musketeers*... [24 July]. Numbers of perfect rosette forms found yesterday [in a case of quartan]. The man saluted, said he was quite well and fit for duty. "Wait a minute, my friend," I said, "you will have a bad attack of fever presently." "Oh, no," he said, "I am quite well." I told him to wait; in an hour his teeth were going like castanets. They now take me for a prophet. I got the mosquitoes on to the two other crescent cases.

You may now feel assured that the "first step" is completely proved. I have tried four cases with identical results.

With kind regards,

Yours truly,

R Ross.

SECUNDERABAD, 30 *July* 1895.

DEAR DR MANSON,

... A very useful way for finding crescents and pigment, suggested by your marginal clot and the mosquito's stomach in which pigment is found almost instantly. Put a large drop of blood on a slide without spreading it out and stir it with a needle and breathe on it for two minutes until it is half dry; then put on the cover glass. The corpuscles are found to be in a viscid yellow mass in which the black pigment of the crescents is seen in a moment. We may thus examine a large quantity of blood in a very small area. This method enabled me to find crescents at once where I had failed after a long study of two ordinary specimens. Useful for diagnosis.*

* Afterwards developed into the "thick-film method."[25]

On 26th. I put three mosquitoes on my quartan. Numbers of intraglobular forms, beautiful rosettes, but no flagellate form seen. (Morning before fever.)

Same day one *flea* on Abdul Wahab. Only four parasites found in the whole insect, which had, however, drunk freely. Two of the parasites (at 40 minutes) were dead spheres and two spent pigment. Crescents were plentiful in mosquitoes (one in a field) the same day. Bugs tried—refused to bite.

... The Patiala affair was opposed by Government for a reason which I am not allowed to mention but which in my opinion is bosh. The fact is that the Indian Government and especially the medical services are utterly ignorant of the importance of this kind of work....

With kind regards.

Yours truly,

R Ross.

Now, after failing to follow the alleged flagellated spores in the mosquito's stomach, I began to adopt quite another procedure. The insects were kept alive for several days after being fed and were then exhaustively searched for any parasites they might contain. If such parasites could be found it would be possible that they might be developed from the motile filaments; and the point could be cleared up by subsequent experiments. I should have to feed mosquitoes on malaria cases as before, keep them for some days, and then examine them exhaustively for any parasites which might be present. On finding a parasite I should have to work out its life history and see if it occurred also in mosquitoes which had not been fed on cases of malaria. Of course this meant an immense study of mosquitoes—because, under the oil-immersion lens, a mosquito appears as big as a hippopotamus is to the naked eye and the object I was looking for need not necessarily be larger in comparison than, say, a nut or an apple, and moreover we had no clue at all as to the position the parasite would take up in the enormous mass of cells of which a mosquito is composed. Nevertheless I now began to attack this object in earnest. It was the method which solved the malaria problem, but it took me two years to find what I sought.

I had already found a parasite in the stegomyia (probably *S scutellaris*) mosquitoes which I had been working with and mentioned the fact in my letter of 10 June (page 42). The objects which I had seen (see figure below) were little barley-shaped sporocysts which were then often called psorosperms or pseudonavicellae and were known to contain the spores of the unicellular parasites called coccidia and gregarines. Accounts of them will be found in the textbooks of Leuckart and of Blanchard of that time. My next letters were full of descriptions of a series of specimens which I was sending to Dr Manson, of various confirmatory observations, of failures to produce malaria in volunteers, etc. It is unnecessary to give this matter and I therefore proceed with extracts regarding the psorosperms or pseudonavicellae, the story of which I now worked out. My next letter describes some specimens which I was sending, especially some stegomyia mosquitoes with crowds of psorosperms in the intestine, and continues:

SECUNDERABAD, 5 *August* 1895.

DEAR DR MANSON,

... Don't you think that these bodies must be looked to very carefully? I have spent the whole week over them. It seems to me that they must still be watched even though they do turn out to be psorosperms. Leuckart and Blanchard say that the sickle-shaped bodies when freed from the psorosperm become amoeboid (as, for instance, the intracorpuscular forms). The bodies appear to be very common among mosquitoes here. I remember finding, however, a much larger form about 20 μm in length with a little rosette near one end. I think that it was in a mosquito which had not been bitten but I have not seen it again. Clearly by your theory it may be present in non-malarialised mosquitoes and yet be connected with the malaria parasite. The bodies appear to me to belong to the sporozoa and to be of a size which we may well imagine the flagella to grow into in a day or two. But you must not be surprised if I go on many a wild goose chase. They certainly appear "encysted and prepared for a lying in wait period."

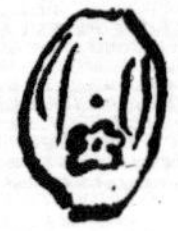

Finding parasites in every case now but no time to *work* at them. Have not a moment leisure from 6.30 am to 8 pm! It is now 7 pm and, barring half an hour for breakfast, I have been at it since 8 am. Luckily feeling fit and full of energy. It takes three hours to hunt through a mosquito; but for my statistics I would throw over examining fresh cases of malaria any more for the present....

With kind regards,

Yours truly,

R Ross.

SECUNDERABAD, 12 *August* 1895.

DEAR DR MANSON,

... I have today got to the bottom of the psorosperms—this *is* what they are. After writing to you I tackled a number of unfed mosquitoes, finding psorosperms in many. I told you that they were in the intestine; but I find by a plate of insects' digestive apparatus in Blanchard that what I thought were the intestines are the malpighian tubes, five of which in the mosquito are inserted into the pylorus. They are long blind tubes consisting of tessellated cells, full of black granules, and easily seen as white threads by the naked eye, as of course you know; and they are present both in larva and pupa. I have now found a way of drawing out the whole apparatus with the ovaries or testicles away from the body cavity so that I can make beautiful specimens, some of which I will send you.* Well, I found the psorosperms in numbers of unfed mosquitoes, mostly at the closed ends of the malpighian tubes where, if they are very numerous, they render the tube friable. I then began to study *grubs*, but found no psorosperms. This morning I took to the pupa, just before hatching into mosquitoes. In the stomach of the first were a number of gregarines of this shape:

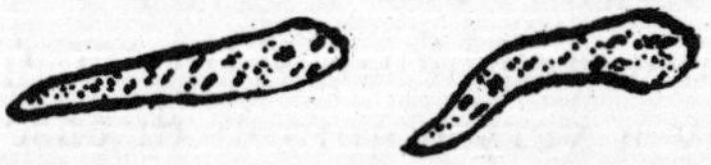

about 100 to 150 μm long, moving rapidly just like slugs, thick end forward. They ceased to move in five minutes. They are full of dark brown granules, but I couldn't see the nucleus. Next I looked at the end of the malpighian tubes—full of large oval bodies about 70 μm long, evidently *encysted gregarines*. On pressure, these and a number of encysting gregarines poured out of the ruptured tubes.

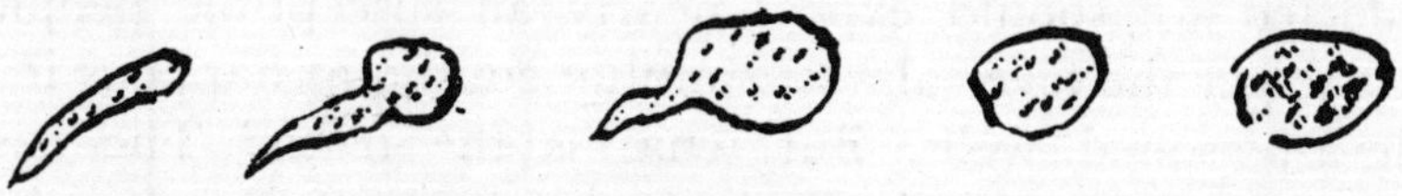

I saw no conjugation forms; the gregarines appear to be single. It was now clear by the *position* of these bodies at the end of the tubes that they were the parents of the psorosperms, but the next pupa put this beyond a doubt by *showing psorosperms inside the encysted gregarines*—so here is the whole chain at once. Now, what do you think? Is it still possible that

* The method of dissecting mosquitoes now in general use. It was published in 1898.[26] For Manson's comment see page 70.

these bodies are another form of the malarial parasite? Please let me have your opinion. So far as I have gone the gregarines live in the pupae, the psorosperms in the mosquitoes. They seem to be hard, encysted little bodies capable of enduring much rough usage and may be discharged either in the faeces or when the insect dies and breaks up. Now the next stage is that of the falciform bodies, which, so far as I can gather from Leuckart and Blanchard, become amoeboid. Is it possible that this amoeboid form is *the intracorpuscular malaria parasite*?

I think, by your original article, that you have had this idea. It is clear in the first place that if the mosquito is the alternative host the malaria parasite must be capable of living in it without man necessarily as an intermediary; we cannot conceive that the insect does no more than carry the parasite from an infected man to drinking water or mud; malaria must be a general endemic disease among mosquitoes; the germ must take only an excursion into man for change of scene and refreshment, so to speak. If this is the case then we must expect the parasite to be a common one among mosquitoes and capable of being propagated from mother to children *ad infinitum* but also capable of rushing off into human beings, probably in its immature form. Such I read your theory to be; and such would probably be the case if the malaria parasite is the amoeboid form of the mosquito's gregarine. These gregarines are evidently a very common disease among mosquitoes in this station; and so far as I can see all the facts which I observe respecting the occurrence of malarial fever here can be explained *best* on the supposition that the poison is conveyed by mosquitoes into *isolated pots of drinking water* in the houses of the men. My reason for this is the following. The whole regiment lives in barracks, or rather huts, about half a mile from a large tank over which the wind blows towards us; the whole regiment drinks water from one large well. Now if the air or well water were infected we should expect nearly all susceptible people in the regiment to get the fever almost simultaneously, as happens in the case of cholera-poisoned wells. But what is the truth? The cases keep dropping in, one or two a day only, out of 700 men. Surely this suggests a most limited and isolated source for the poison, such in fact as the infection of a chatty or two of drinking water in the men's huts by ripe, infected mosquitoes. The mosquitoes themselves of course may come from the tank and it is thus that lakes and marshes have got the reputation of being malarious; but so far as I can see the poison, however general it may be in a district, must be absorbed from very localised and not general sources in order to explain the scanty and successive, and not general and simultaneous, occurrences of cases of fever (interesting errors!).

On the whole, then, I think these gregarines fall in wonderfully well with your ideas of the alternative form. Even if they are not the malaria parasite I can't help thinking that they will be found to have some human pathological import because, as you say, men and mosquitoes fall exactly into the usual parasitological circle. The question is, what do the free flagella develop into? Why not straight into young gregarines? I have not observed gregarines in malarialised mosquitoes, but I may easily have mistaken them for normal cells because I would not have recognised them today if I had not seen them crawling about, which they ceased to do in a few minutes. Then again, the gregarines I have seen must have entered the young grubs because they were fully developed in the pupa. Do you think that it is possible for them to enter the mature insect by way of human blood and develop into psorosperms before its death? Why not? I will look very closely. I must also try to find gregarines in the grubs and must see how the psorosperms leave the mosquito, whether by the intestine or only after death. I am certain too that I once saw a much larger kind of psorosperm, I believe in an unfed mosquito (don't remember).

You can imagine my excitement over all this—though it may turn out to be a wrong scent. My work is tremendous—I have *twenty* malaria cases in hospital—can't possibly work at them properly....

13 August. Gregarines found in two more pupa and in a number of larvae, down to small ones but not down to the smallest size yet. Encysting gregarines in one old larva. They occur also in the intestine. Nuclei often clearly made out. By oil-immersion the granules are seen in continual motion and a sort of bubble forms at the creature's big end [drawing]. Granules at tail bigger than the rest. Clear double contour. Length measured by micrometer 200 μm for about the largest size and 100 μm or less for the smallest. The youngest grubs contain the smallest gregarines....

With kind regards,

Yours truly,

R Ross.

SECUNDERABAD, 20 *August* 1895.

DEAR DR MANSON,

... Having worked out the connection between the gregarines and psorosperms, the next thing to do was to find how the latter left the insect and how far they mature within it. Though gregarines are to be found in almost every grub, I have often failed in finding psorosperms in mature mosquitoes. Hence, if I had not overlooked them, I concluded they must pass out during life. I examined a number of unfed mosquitoes which had died naturally—no psorosperms; then a number of fed mosquitoes at two, three, four, and five days—only a few psorosperms occasionally. On the other hand they were often plentiful in newly hatched mosquitoes; in one I found a single *gregarine*, in two others cysts full of psorosperms; hence it is probable that they pass out about the second day after hatching, but how I cannot make out; I cannot find any in stomach, intestines, or about the anus.

At the same time I examined water at the bottom of the bottle in which mosquitoes were kept—no psorosperms to be found. I looked at eggs which had been laid—same result. On considering large numbers of gregarines in grubs and pupae and often small numbers of psorosperms in even newly hatched mosquitoes I began to think that they were got rid of during pupa stage. I looked accordingly at the *cast off skin of pupae—numbers of psorosperms*. This fact is always confirmed by examinations up to today so that this at least is one way in which the psorosperms pass out, though I can't imagine how they get from the blind end of the malpighian tubes to the skin. They are most numerous generally in the head-piece of the pupa pelt and are seen as numerous hard little bodies with a collection of granules at one part....

[21 August].... Not a man doing microscopic malaria diagnosis in the whole presidency yet, so far as I know; the science not taught at Madras medical schools (of course every hospital assistant ought to be able to find the parasite); microscopes not supplied; no official circulars on the subject; no reply yet about your charts.... The fact is that by some fatuity the worst men rise to the top of the service here—that is, the so-called smart men, the regulation-wallers [*sic*] never the scientific men. Why was not V Carter made Surgeon General?...

With kind regards believe me,

Yours truly,

R Ross.

SECUNDERABAD, 31 *August* 1985.

DEAR DR MANSON,

I was obliged to miss the last post owing to being suddenly engaged in a medicolegal case. It lasted from morning to night for three days; 100 rupees a day, but forced me to waste some malarialised mosquitoes I wished to examine....

As I told you, the gregarines encyst in the pupa stage, and the psorosperms are mature and discharged *by the bowel* at the end of the pupa stage and the first days of the imago stage. I have now frequently seen psorosperms in stomach, intestine, and about the anus. It appears that the gregarine cysts break up in position (that is, in the ends of the malpighian tubes), so that the psorosperms are passed out entirely free and are found free in large numbers in the malpighian tubes themselves. The cast-off skins of the pupae often contain numbers of psorosperms, as I said, but still numbers are carried away by the flying insect and evidently scattered abroad through its bowel as it flies. Thus I caught a mosquito which was trying to bite me; a stream of psorosperms was issuing from its anus and could be traced up the intestine, the stomach, and the malpighian tubes. I have kept psorosperms in water for a fortnight now but have not observed any change. The psorosperms themselves show certain differences which I will work at. They are seldom to be found, I think, in old insects, either fed or unfed, and seem to be almost always got rid of before death. In order to find psorosperms in pupa pelts it is necessary to separate the pupa from the larvae because the latter have the habit of sucking the cast-off skins, evidently for the numbers of infusoria and amoebae, etc which they contain; in this process the psorosperms are shaken out and sink to the bottom of the vessel, being *heavier than water*, or *are swallowed by the larvae*. If, however, the pupa is put in a bottle by itself, the skin is generally found full of psorosperms and so is the digestive apparatus of the living insect which has emerged.

I think these are facts as I have worked long and hard at the various points. The upshot is that the psorosperms must be discharged into two *different worlds* as it were; some are left in the water in which the grub lived and others are scattered—where? Now I will reason in the way you have taught me to. Suppose that the psorosperms were meant *only* to infect mosquito grubs, or perhaps some kind of fish or water insect, would not the gregarines *make haste* to complete their development in time to allow of all the psorosperms being discharged into the water in which the grub lived; or would they not *retard* their development in order to allow the discharge to take place *when the eggs are laid*? But as a fact most of them are got rid of just at a time when the insect is *farthest* from water and is busy *hovering round men*. It is indeed almost certain that *while the insect is biting* it is discharging psorosperms upon the human skin which may be directly conveyed to the mouth by the man scratching himself and then accidently sucking his finger. How does this look? Or the psorosperms may be simply scattered over a sleeper's mouth.

I must say that this psorosperm theory is looking very promising, especially this latest development of it, which I have been driven to by hard facts. Nature would, I apprehend, scarcely waste the psorosperms by causing them to be evacuated just at the moment when the insect is farthest from the water—that is supposing they are meant only for grubs or water animals. In short, I believe that the psorosperms are *meant for men*, as well as for reinfecting the grubs of course; hence their being discharged into *two worlds*. But what disease can they possibly cause? Not dysentery I suppose; malaria seems the only supposition. Well, I have got three tubes containing psorosperms and I hope to give each of these tubes to a man tomorrow, but I must begin with small doses of psorosperms—so you must not be disappointed if I fail at first.

1 September, Sunday. The contents of three tubes given to three healthy young men at 8.45 this morning. Each tube contained psorosperms from the insects (direct from the malpighian tubes). One contained a pupa pelt. All given in water by mouth. If the experiments fail I will try spraying the psorosperms into the lungs....

The nature of the experiment was fully explained in the presence of witnesses to all the men who submitted to it.

I have a sort of feeling that it will be successful and, as you will readily understand, a kind of religious excitement over it. God knows what will be the result. If the experiment fails I shall have to take a holiday because the work and excitement are telling upon me; but I shall soon begin work again on other lines. I feel convinced it is the mosquito....

3rd. Holiday today (only the sick of three regiments, one court marshall [sic], and a medical board).... In this station there are about a dozen doctors, not one of whom possesses an oil-immersion or works at malaria. Is this to go on for ever? Yet Laveran's discovery is essential to treatment. I have just been adding up my results for four months. I have recorded 110 cases (ague or simple continued fever). Out of these I have found the parasite in 65, or 59%, having missed it in numbers of other cases simply owing to pressure of work, I expect.... Now is not the apathy of the heads of the department quite monstrous? It amounts to a national scandal. Why don't they supply proper microscopes and make their men work at the subject? Why don't they teach it in medical schools? In districts where fever is prevalent why don't they have the fever investigated by the microscope? Really if nothing is done soon there will be a scandal. The fact is that our surgeons general don't seem to recognise their positions or their duties in respect to new scientific discoveries. It is the same with *Amoeba coli*.... Moreover, qualified men should be sent round the country to teach—Laveranity apostles. Oil-immersions ought to be supplied at once.... I have examined the stomach, intestine, kidneys, and ovaries of three malarialised mosquitoes pretty carefully but have seen nothing which I can swear are parasites. They were killed at three and four days. If the psorosperms fail I must of course work entirely in this direction. But except the psorosperms I have seen nothing yet which looks sufficiently hard and encysted to withstand *out of door* life. The hitch in the psorosperm theory comes in when we inquire what the flagella develop into. Is it possible too that a single animal can undergo so many metamorphoses? I am looking forward anxiously to your opinion of it all.

With kind regards,

Yours truly,

R Ross.

I have given my work and thoughts on this gregarine parasite of the mosquito at some length because of its interest. In our stage of knowledge at that time my conjectures that it might be the mosquito stage of the malaria parasite were quite reasonable and the matter had to be worked out experimentally down to the fullest detail. It is the method of "trial by error" which is often the only method that can lead to success in the solution of many problems, including mathematical ones; and it will be seen later that I had to pursue the same method for every organism which I found in the insects. Really the great objection to the gregarine theory was contained in the penultimate sentence of the last letter. I had found the complete cycle of the gregarines and there was no room left, according to general parasitological knowledge, for another cycle consisting of the malaria parasite to be interpolated.

But I now perceived that my hypothesis was beginning to run away with me a little and that I must take time to give my mind a rest. I therefore intended to attempt to follow the flagellated spores again as suggested at the end of my letter of 18 July. For this purpose I proposed to mix the blood contained in the mosquito's stomach with a little salt solution, with or without stain, so that the whole contents of the said blood might be spread out evenly under the microscope, enabling me to follow the flagella exactly. If I had done this I would have anticipated MacCallum and Opie in their fine discovery made two years later and would no doubt have actually seen that the flagella are sperms. In fact I came very near this discovery in my letter of 18 July, describing the "adventures" of one. But unfortunately, just after writing the letter last recorded I received orders to proceed forthwith to Bangalore.

During this period other things were done. Being a convert, like St Paul, I became a militant apostle. Surgeon Colonel Lawrie was then the head of the medical services of the Nizam of Hyderabad and lived at Chudderghat, near Secunderabad. He was a very capable man, a brilliant surgeon, and the organiser of one of the finest medical schools in India—direct, energetic, and witty. But he did not believe in "Laveranity" because, in fact, one of his officers had made the mistake which I had previously alluded to of taking artifacts for malaria parasites. I gathered that he detected the error and, like myself, therefore disbelieved in the whole business. But he carried his scepticism too far and did not know enough about the blood to recognise that the real Laveran bodies were indeed parasites. I had an amusing controversy with him in a paper which I published later[27] and a still more amusing interview at which I suffered a crushing defeat (page 95).

4

The Scavengers. Bangalore, 1895–1897

My transfer to Bangalore on special sanitary duty was the first of the three serious interruptions from which my malaria work suffered, all of which by some evil fatality occurred just at the moments when rapid advances seemed to be assured. But unlike the two later interruptions, this first one was justified by the event because it gave me an almost unique experience in practical sanitation which was invaluable when we came after 1898 to apply the proved mosquito-malaria theory for the benefit of suffering humanity.

The civil and military station of Bangalore was an island of territory ruled directly by the Government of India within the dominions of the Maharaja of Mysore. It was under the jurisdiction of the British Resident at the court of the Maharaja and contained (1) the military garrison under the General Commanding and (2) the civil population of about 90 000 people under the Bangalore Municipal Commission. On previous occasions my post of staff surgeon at Bangalore was connected with the garrison, but I was now sent for by the resident (then Mr Lee Warner, Indian Civil Service) in connection with the affairs of the civil population and the municipality. The occasion was this. For a long time that capable officer, Surgeon Lieut Colonel A F Dobson, MB, Indian Medical Service, who was then residency surgeon (that is, the medical officer to the resident, the civil staff, and the Bowring Civil Hospital), had been much dissatisfied with the sanitary administration of the municipality. The native quarter was in a filthy condition and was frequently swept by epidemics, especially of cholera. Now in August 1895 another outbreak of cholera was beginning and he considered that the municipality was not working hard enough or wisely enough to check it. There was a small sanitary board consisting of the Principal Medical Officer of the troops, Surgeon Colonel S B Hunt, Army Medical Service, the president, Dr Dobson, the secretary, and a junior military officer; and this board complained to the resident, especially in letter No 651 of 11 September, and advised a complete reorganisation of the sanitary affairs of the municipality, then consisting of about 20 elected native members and six ex officio members (mostly British) under an Indian civilian as chairman (then Mr A M Slight—an excellent young man). But as no reform was likely to occur within this municipality itself Dobson advised Mr Lee Warner to ask the Government of India for my services, partly to deal with the cholera and partly to report on the sanitary condition of the station in general. It was rather a miracle, I think, that this request was acceded to, even though I held a Diploma of Public Health. But I received my orders, closed the malaria investigation for a time, packed up my few belongings, and arrived in Bangalore on 9 September 1895.

On my arrival I received the most astonishingly ample and indeed dictatorial powers. These were: "To direct and enforce the sanitary operations conducted by the municipality in consultation with the residency surgeon. To submit a report to the resident on the present state of affairs.... To examine thoroughly the constitution of the sanitary department and to suggest in full detail the changes needed to improve its efficiency.... To deal specially in your report with the following matters, etc." Seldom has a mere doctor been given such powers, and I availed myself of them. Taking up my residence in a tent in the compound of the West End Hotel, I was given a carriage for my use day and night, a clerk, sanitary inspectors, and peons. In two days, in consultation with Dobson, I sent the municipality an ultimatum regarding measures which they were neglecting and followed this by numerous similar documents, while every hour I rushed off to see the cases of cholera scattered over the station. Within five weeks I sent the resident six emergency reports and extracted 5000 rupees from the municipality for the necessary work! There were 20 deaths from cholera in August, 64 in September, seven in October, and then the epidemic ceased and I set about the general sanitary investigation. My full report to the resident (Residency Press, Bangalore) was submitted on 20 January 1896 and contains 126 printed foolscap pages dealing with the whole subject (and is, I am told, still in use).

From 18 January 1896 I was appointed, professedly under the municipality but really under the resident, to carry out the difficult task of giving effect to my own recommendations and on 26 May 1896 I became officiating residency surgeon, while Dr Dobson went home on furlough. On 29 March 1897 I took leave to Ootacamund pending Dobson's return from furlough, thus ending my arduous but agreeable duties at Bangalore. I had been there for 18 months. Soon after I arrived Mr Lee Warner had been succeeded at the residency by Mr Mackworth Young, ICS, who in turn was followed by Colonel D Robertson. After I left Bangalore the last-named published the following order dated 7 April 1897—of which I am very proud: "Surgeon Major Ross," he said, "having left Bangalore, the resident desires to place on record his high appreciation of the services rendered by this officer.... Surgeon Major Ross's interesting and exhaustive report on 'Cholera, General Sanitation, and the Sanitary Department and Regulations in the Civil and Military Station of Bangalore' was received in January 1896, and in reviewing it Mr Mackworth Young, the late resident, remarked that Dr Ross had 'discharged the duty entrusted to him in a most able and efficient manner,' and he requested that his best thanks might be conveyed 'for his excellent report, which will contribute largely to the welfare of the station.' The main principles of that report were accepted by the municipal commissioners, who were so assured of the soundness of the advice offered by Surgeon Major Ross that they applied for his services in order that he might initiate the reforms advocated by him and set in order their sanitary department. In the execution of his various and important duties Surgeon Major Ross has never spared himself. His work throughout, in which a large measure of success has been attained, has been remarkable for the zeal, thoroughness, and tact displayed, and the resident is confident that for this work no more capable officer could have been selected." Copies of this were sent to the Foreign Department of the Government of India and to the Surgeon General with the Government of Madras. But I have never been employed again by my countrymen on this kind of service.

I have no space for details. We had to revise the whole system of conservancy and refuse removal, the latrine system, the surface drainage, and even taxation and the municipal regulations and by-laws and to institute a municipal laboratory, registration of vendors of food, milk, and water, and a hundred other improvements. From January 1896 I was an ex officio member of the municipality and, with the continual and effective support of Surgeon Colonel Dobson, carried through measure after measure, often against strong opposition. The list comprises no less than 58 proposals, resolutions, or rejections! Since then

I have always been very sceptical regarding the worth of all councils, committees, and public assemblies. Most of the members, both European and native, were "guinea-pigs"—that is, persons who knew nothing of the business on hand and were too lazy to learn and who, when they were required to vote, would look furtively round the tables to see how the majority were likely to vote; and their opinion was absolutely worthless. A few were practising oratory at the expense of the others and some were trying to be professional politicians—that is, persons who cared nothing for the rightness of policy but everything for the effect of their speeches when reported in the local press. I tried to persuade these humbugs to go round their wards with me in order to see the dirt, squalor, and ill health of the people—they were, of course, always so sorry that they were otherwise engaged. The leader of the "opposition" was a retired English engineer who was very angry because he was not allowed to put his finger in the sanitary pie; and the measure of ours which caused the most "popular indignation" was my cess tax, a small payment for the daily removal of ordure, which the ingenuous householders used previously to keep for weeks in their houses in order to sell it to contractors for manure. The papers also attacked me for this "imposition" and I received abusive anonymous letters about it. One said, "Have you no sense you fool? Shame, shame, shame!" On the other hand several of the commissioners were admirable persons, especially Mr Abdur Rahman (I think), a magistrate, and Mr Annasawawmy Mudaliar, who was not only as good a speaker (in English) as I have ever heard but who often accompanied me in my rounds, studied my proposals, and persuaded his poor people to adopt them—a Hindu who possessed every virtue of a Christian gentleman. I also received much help from Captain A C Joly de Lotbinière, RE, who was engaged in providing a piped water supply for the town; and Mr Slight, the president, though he was criticised by Dobson, always tried to help us. On the whole we had nothing to complain about, for we passed almost every measure we wanted and I am sure that all my "enemies" were also my friends.

The street gutters of the native quarter were really shocking, as they ran with sewage, and I therefore devised some new patterns and described them in a *Memorandum on Open Sewage Drains* which was published by the municipality on 24 September 1896. They were tried in a slum in South Blackpully and it was interesting to watch how the whole quarter was improved by this means—the householders mended their walls, doors, and yards in emulation.

Our sanitary reforms were not likely to be immediately effective and we had three outbreaks of cholera during 1916. As usual, the disease began to creep up from the east coast in April and I posted hospital assistants at railway stations and crossroads to intercept cases, disinfected wells, and instituted a system of rewards to our sweepers and scavengers and other for reporting cases (the politicians of the municipality accused me of paying spies to watch the householders!). On 4 June a case got through into the town and on the 14th and subsequently 27 cases were reported close together. I saw by my "spot map" that they were all probably infected from the same public well and closed it on the 14th. The epidemic ceased by 20 June. On 15 July, however, it commenced again in another part of the town but was again suppressed there after a fortnight by active disinfection of all the wells and closing of the most suspected ones. We had scarcely begun to congratulate ourselves on this result when, on 8 August, a terrible epidemic began in the worst parts of the town called North Blackpully and the East General Bazaar—areas swarming with slums and containing about 20000 of the poorest people. There were 582 wells here within a space of about one-quarter of a mile square, most of them within private tenements where we could not easily touch them owing to "caste prejudices"—that is, gross superstitions. We did what we could. We closed the wells in batches; we disinfected them over and over again; we told the people to boil their drinking water and provided it ourselves; we gave them hot coffee and medicine early in the morning; we disinfected backyards, drains, and rooms occupied by the dying. All in vain. The Angel of Death had descended among them and smote the poor wretches right and left. They died within 12 hours. Secondary cases were numerous: where the child died today, the mother or father would be dead tomorrow. The people, usually so patient and good, were stricken with terror, cried to their gods, formed processions, and glared at those who tried to help them; and the heavy rain washed the reeking filth of the streets and latrines into the shallow poison-pools they called wells. It was a dreadful time. We could do nothing more. Either the cholera vibrio had got into some source of water which we failed to find and close or it had penetrated into the whole subsoil water of the locality. Then suddenly, as usual after about a month, the pestilence cleared and vanished like an evil thunderstorm. But 219 cases were reported during that time, of which about 150 died; and probably very many of the cases and deaths were not reported at all in the final rush and terror.

I should like to take the politicians who so often belittle and neglect sanitation and medical science—I should like to take them by the scruff of the neck and fling them into the midst of an Indian outbreak of cholera and into the midst of the filth and dirt which their bad laws and feeble administration allow to continue! I am not talking of British politicians only but of Indian politicians, such as municipal commissioners, as well—they are all alike. In this case they had allowed these slums to grow up during years of neglect; every house had its poison-pool and science could do nothing.

Yet 16 years had elapsed since Robert Koch had discovered the cause of cholera. Unfortunately certain "eminent scientists" would not believe him and one of these was the official investigator of the Indian Government. The world still fails to recognise that Tom, Dick, and Harry are not necessarily good scientific investigators. Often they do not possess the brains either to make sound discoveries themselves or even to understand them when made by others. They can pass examinations, write textbooks, and become "eminent scientists," it is true; but the real investigator, like the real poet, is born, not made. Now governments love to appoint Tom, Dick, and Harry to their most important scientific posts and then look upon them as being true prophets. One might as well try to establish a college of poets out of a band of literary journalistic critics; and thus it was that India neglected Koch's discovery all those years. Now, however, in 1896 a revolution was beginning. Koch's work had been proved completely and Mr E H Hankin, Chemical Examiner at Agra, had been following it up by finding the vibrio in cholera-infected food and water and by showing how to disinfect wells by permanganate of potash. Also Mr W M W Haffkine had arrived in India (in 1893) from the Pasteur Institute bringing with him his famous anticholera vaccine and was now trying it in India on a large scale—and he laughed at the hypercritical criticism of the Indian authorities. Thus things were now beginning to move in India at last. But while I was able to employ Hankin's disinfection of wells at Bangalore, I was not able to use Haffkine's vaccine because my laboratory and staff were not nearly developed enough to give it to large numbers of people, while the people themselves would have objected in those days. During the 16 years' neglect of Koch's discovery about eight million Indians had died of cholera; and I may add that there was enough prima facie evidence of the discovery to have justified extensive work on the subject from 1880 onwards.

These epidemics were reported by me to the resident in two letters dated 8 July and 29 September 1896 and I was much distressed at our failure to check the last outbreak. The following rough verses occur in one of my *In Exile* notebooks:

Twice have I driven thee hence,
  Defeated, dreadful Guest—
O murderous Pestilence:
  This time thou conquerest.

Loudly the people's cry
  To thee in prayer swells;
I seek to purify
  The deadly poisoned wells—

In vain. The languid child
  Lies on his mother's knee;
The mother follows; wild
  The people shriek to thee.

On one occasion I tracked a source of infection to a well-to-do milkman who had kept the best and cleanest cowhouse in the station. I charged him with having a case of cholera. He denied it but just as I was leaving I saw a movement under some clothing cast in a corner. It was his little daughter dying of cholera.

But the abiding questions were those of general sanitation. On 17 February 1896 I went to Poona to inspect the admirable system of poudrette manufacture which had been installed there for years by a most energetic and capable native member of the municipality and later we adopted his method, with some simplifications, at Bangalore. Thence I went on to Bombay to study many sanitary details there. It was just before the terrible Indian outbreak of plague had commenced in the city, though even then there were rumours of it, and the case was another instance of want of scientific study and preparation by the Indian authorities. On the way back I spent a day (23 February) at Khandala, on the ghats, in order to see the great caves and their carvings.

Above all it was necessary to organise refuse removal on the cheapest and most efficient basis possible (there were no house sewers), and day after day I accompanied the scavengers and sweepers in their early and disgusting work—sometimes rising before daybreak to do so—in order to learn exactly how an Indian city was to be kept clean and what improvements should be made. These experiences are not easily forgotten—the glorious stars glittering in the chill morning wind, the murky lanterns, the clinking pails, the patient oxen, the awful stenches. And the poor men themselves, the last pariahs and outcasts of society, toiling while others slept; and yet, in a way, the civilisation of the thronged cities was based upon their labour. Thank heaven I was able to increase their pay and give them good lanterns at least.

Great is sanitation—the greatest work except discovery, I think, that a man can do. Here is a city seething with filth and disease. What is the use of preaching high moralities, philosophies, policies, and arts to people who dwell in these appalling slums—sometimes whole families of them crowded into one cell, mixed with cattle, vermin, and ordure? Your job, sanitarian, is plain! You must wipe away those slums, that filth, these diseases. You shall work in the darkness while others sleep. None shall know of your labour, no one shall thank you, you shall die forgotten. The great ones of the earth shall despise you, shall hamper you, shall even punish you. The lofty rulers of the world shall not deign even to look at you but shall prate of gods and virtues, liberties and laws, and shall busy themselves pouring the wine of wealth from one vessel into another, drinking much by the way and spilling more! But you, O cleanser, shall always be a pariah. Fret not, however; for these dying children shall live, and some day this hideous slum shall become a city of gardens and it is you who will have done it.

We shall reach the higher civilisation not by any of the politicians' shibboleths, methods of government, manners of voting, liberty, self determination, and the rest, all of which have failed—but first by the scientific ordering of cities until they are fit for men of the higher civilisation to dwell in. We must begin by being cleansers. I find the following two stanzas in my notebooks:

> "Ascend," the Prelate cries,
> "From Men to angels." "Then,
> First learn," the Sage replies,
> "To grow from Apes to Men";

and also

> We cry, "God, make us Kings,
> Poets or Prophets here!"
> The scornful Answer rings,
> "First be My Scavenger."

Of course, owing to the great pressure of my sanitary work I was unable to continue my malaria researches for months after my arrival in Bangalore in 1895. But I continued to write letters to Manson from time to time. My first one from Bangalore was dated 18 September and in this I told him the results of my experiments in which I gave psorosperms to three young men. All of them had slight reactions and I wrote: "The two cases were like Lutchman's and I think that the psorosperms bring on some reaction, *probably malarial*. The cases struck me as malarial due to insufficient doses. Will try 3000 psorosperms next time ... a fresh cholera case and must be off at once ... have plenary powers to reform all sanitary details." In his reply of 9 September Manson was very doubtful about the theory that psorosperms are connected with malaria but added, "still it is necessary to clear the ground of *Gregarina culicidis* and you do right to get clear conceptions on this point before going further." I wrote to him on 4 October: "I am of course not sure as to the result of my experiments of 1 September, but two of the men certainly got something like malarial fever of a very slight kind; my only conclusion is that psorosperms cause some kind of reaction, query what kind? Further experiment, however, may still prove me to be mistaken. Now about some points of your objections." I told him that I had failed to infect young mosquito larvae which had lived in water full of psorosperms and doubted whether the whole history between the psorosperm and the young gregarine was fully known yet. On the other hand I thought "it would indeed be very curious if the same parasite were capable of going through two separate life cycles.... I admit all the difficulties, especially about the flagella, and don't presume even to put forward a gregarine theory, but it is curious that (as I believe I haven't told you) I could find gregarines only in the mosquitoes at Begumpett (my regiment's quarters), the most feverish locality in Secunderabad. Just before leaving Secunderabad for this place I examined five or six batches of grubs from other parts—no gregarines at all! Then again after I suppressed the gregarine-bearing mosquitoes at Begumpett on 22 August there appears to have been scarcely any more fever in the regiment.... 8 October. The difficulty, if the malarial parasite in the mosquito is like what it is in man, will lie in distinguishing it from the nuclei of cells. I have seen so many things like malaria parasites in the mosquito and in the grub, but I have a lot to learn about their anatomy." I then gave Manson a summary of the cases of malaria in which I had found parasites in Secunderabad. They were: "112 fever cases; 21 spring tertians; 38 summer-autumns; 2 quartans; 3 mixed; 5 doubtful; 69 total parasites found." In the rest of my letter I described my work in Bangalore and remarked, "I tell you privately I have been credited, perhaps by a silly slip of the pen, with almost unlimited power and I have seized upon the order (or mistake) and immediately *commanded* the municipality to make three great reforms. Dobson is at my back.... I have acted with such celerity that the astonished president of the municipality ... has conceded my provisional demands and has allowed me actually to carry my reforms half through before he or the resident or anyone understands the tyrannical nature of my action."

Shortly after arrival in Bangalore in September 1895 I found that my wife could join me there and she arrived in Madras about 23 November with our three children and their nurse, Miss Agnes Carrington. On 26 November 1895 I wrote to Manson: "I went down to Madras, however, to meet my wife, who has arrived with the children from England, and I took the opportunity of showing them all (ie the doctors) the malaria parasite and now they are at it keenly, especially a man called Sturmer, who writes me that he has found the parasite in five out of nine cases already. I showed them a triple quartan and a summer-autumn, the latter occurring in a case of elephantiasis which a man showed me in order to catch me, thinking that he had elephantoid fever. The laugh was turned against him.... My labour has been frightful—working from 6.30 am to 11.30 and 12 at night.... I have not been able to find any psorosperms here or in Madras.... I enclose a letter from Sturmer to me which will show you how keen he is.... None of them in Madras were able to find the animal till I went down there. But I saw Cleghorn [the Director General, Indian Medical Service] in Madras and spoke about malaria. Everything is now merely a question of want of time with me; there are only 24 hours in a day. I reported about mosquito investigations to Government in response to a circular which Cleghorn sent round."

Manson's replies deal chiefly with his studies of the specimens which I had sent to him and with requests for more specimens. He did not seem to be much interested in Bangalore sanitation! With reference to my method of finding crescents (page 50) he remarked in his of 9 September: "I like your dodge of finding crescents and shall try it in the first case I get. It ought to answer with other pigmented forms as well and should prove a great gain in diagnosis. If it comes out all right I shall send the part of your letter referring to this to the *BMJ*, adding that I have tried it and find it good." On 21 October 1895 he wrote to me regarding my method of dissecting mosquitoes (page 53): "How do you manage to get the alimentary canal out so perfectly without injury to malpighian tubes and other delicate structures?" Both of us were much alive to the possibility of other workers stepping in very soon to complete my interrupted work on the mosquito theory, and indeed on 26 July 1895 Manson had already written about the theory, "the Frenchies and Italians will pooh-pooh it at first, then adopt it, and then claim it as their own. See if they don't. But push on with it and don't let them forestall you. They won't have time this autumn and they will not have a chance to work seriously at the matter till next June or so. You have got a year ahead of them and in that time you should have solved the problem in its principles at all events. Leave the details for them to work out, which they will do well and with much wrangling." As a matter of fact they did not begin on the work until *three* years later—that is, in the summer of 1898, after I had solved the problem; and the difficulties were much greater than Manson supposed.

Even in the midst of my very hard sanitary work I found time to search for malaria cases at the Bowring Civil Hospital. On 4 December 1895 I wrote to Manson saying that I had a good case of crescents and was trying mosquitoes again; and I then added that I was "inclined to claim discovery of a new species of malaria parasite—namely, the eye forms (page 48). Found two cases, one of dysentery and fever, the other fever, with numbers of these. They are certainly living creatures and are motile to a small extent but not amoeboid. Are they young crescents?" I think this was nearly the last time I was deceived by these bodies as some months afterwards I found numbers of them in my own blood and in that of other healthy persons. They deluded numerous observers and I remember that one writer claimed them as the cause of fever in Palestine. They are probably micrococci from the skin which fall into the red corpuscles when the specimen is made.

In my letter to Manson of 12 December I apologised for not sending all the specimens which he had asked for so frequently. He wanted mosquitoes fed on malaria cases and preserved in glycerin or formalin; but, already overworked as I was, it was a very serious matter for me to obtain them because I had first to hunt for malaria cases through the station and then to try and get the mosquitoes to bite. At the same time I was sure that he would not be able to get good results from sectioned mosquitoes "for the simple mathematical reason—namely, that unless the blood is swarming with parasites you won't find more than one or two in a whole section." I always felt also, though I did not like to say so, that he could have done the work in London almost as easily as I had done it in Secunderabad. I was wasting what little time I had to spare.

My letters of 29 January, 26 February, 25 March, 5 April, 26 April, and 27 May 1896 record only want of time to do much malaria work; but during that period I tried to infect some more men with psorosperms, giving 19 experiments altogether. What really made me sceptical was a fact noted in mine of 25 March: "By the by, I have entirely forgotten to tell you up to date that I myself took some psorosperms in October and again in December—no result at all. I took about 1500 and 2000 on the two occasions; but then I have never had fever though I have been in malarious places. Three days after the second dose I thought I felt ill, but it was probably liver." And when such cases failed entirely I thought that I had done enough in this line and began to consider whether some other route of infection was not possible. Thus on 27 May I wrote to Manson: "None of the experimental cases have come in yet and all look like being failures. The last case appeared to be looking ill after 48 hours, but it passed off next day and he has been well ever since. The psorosperms were given at all degrees of freshness and in large numbers, so it certainly looks, as it was to be suspected, that they are not the thing. But I will watch and pray and try a few more experiments; ... but the belief is growing on me that the disease is communicated by the bite of the mosquito. What do you think? She always injects a small quantity of fluid with her bite—what if the parasites get into the system in this manner? I shall experiment in this direction and shall also dissect the head." *This in fact proved to be the case.* See Manson's opinion, page 74.

During this period, however, I tried to push the study of the parasites and told Manson on 26 February: "I preached Laveranity at Poona and Bombay, making one convert in the former ... a young chap called Kilkelly, IMS; saw the Parsee doctor Surveyor, whom you knew in Bombay, and showed him a spring tertian; and also saw some relapsing fever 'spirilla.' Do you know I believe it is an *animal parasite*, some possible connection with surra (?)—hardly possible, but it does not look like bacteria. The Bombay men don't care a rush for the malaria parasite; they won't take the trouble to look at my spring tertian. Madras men are waking up well." In fact Dr Sturmer, IMS, whom I have mentioned before and who was one of the district medical officers in Madras, came to Bangalore during Christmas 1895 to work with me; and in January I made many demonstrations to Captain Carr White, IMS, who had succeeded me in the staff surgeoncy at Bangalore and who wrote a paper confirming my results in the *Indian Medical Gazette*, April 1896.

All this time we had been living at the West End Hotel, but in the hot weather I sent my family to the Farringdon Hotel, Ootacamund, and myself took a few days' leave there—which was all the leave I had during during that year. On a second occasion I was called back prematurely by the outbreak of cholera already described. When the rains began my family returned to Bangalore and we all lived in Surgeon Colonel Dobson's house on the high ground, he and Mrs Dobson having gone to England on furlough; and we stayed there till I left Bangalore finally in 1897.

I was not able to do much malaria work until September 1896, but as Dr Dobson had left for home I was then in charge of the Bowring Civil Hospital. I began at once by testing experimentally the hypothesis which I mentioned to Manson in my letter of 27 May—namely, that malaria may be communicated by the bites of mosquitoes and not, as Manson thought, by people swallowing water in which infected mosquitoes had died.

A number of mosquitoes, all bred from larvae in captivity and of all the kinds which I could collect (many specimens of brindled and grey mosquitoes), were fed upon several patients with numerous parasites in their blood. One of these patients had all three kinds of parasite in him and I specially employed this case, as well as many varieties of mosquito, in order to increase the chances of one at least of the species of mosquito present being appropriate for one at least of the species of parasite. After feeding, the insects were kept alive for one or two days and were then applied in considerable numbers on two occasions to Mr K N Appia, assistant surgeon of the Bowring Civil Hospital at Bangalore, who courageously volunteered for the experiment. Mr Appia had suffered from malarial fever some years previously but not since then, so that if he should be attacked by fever shortly after the experiment it would be strong evidence, if not proof, in favour of the inoculation theory. He remained, however, absolutely free from fever. He was then bitten by five mosquitoes which had been partially fed *immediately before* on a case of crescents—on the supposition that the insects may carry the infection mechanically, as the tsetse-fly carries nagana; but the result was again negative. Lastly two other individuals were bitten by mosquitoes fed from three to five days previously; still without effect. I judged, then, either that infection is not produced in this way, or that the proper species of mosquito had not been employed, or that they had not been kept for the proper period after feeding; and I proposed to return to the subject again.

These experiments were reported to Manson in my letter to him of 21 September 1896, and full descriptions of them and of the previous experiments on men with water containing dead mosquitoes or psorosperms were published in December 1896.[28] My ultimate conclusion was given in this paper as follows: "On the whole then, I think, I am justified in saying this much: that while we cannot dream of stating definitely on the strength of these experiments that there is something connected with the mosquitoes which is capable of imparting fever, the three positive results are still curious and tend to be in favour of the truth of Manson's theory." Of course I had to give considerably increased rewards if the subjects of the experiments got any fever and many of us thought and think that some Indians are clever enough to get fever whenever they like; and my ultimate conclusion was that the apparently successful cases which I had obtained were probably of this nature. Anyway the facts stand as I stated them. Perhaps also the psorosperms do really cause some reaction in human beings, although we now know that they are not in any way connected with malaria.

All this time Manson had been disturbed at what he evidently thought were my sanitary divagations and on 20 May 1896 had written: "It seems to me a great misfortune that the best men in your service are the hardest worked, that is to say that their energies and abilities are directed into such base utilitarian channels as practical sanitation of cities and the charge of big establishments requiring more administrative ability than brains." I did not agree with this view at all. To me it always seemed that the practical application is the summit of all biological research. I did not undertake this work on malaria in the interests of zoology but in the interests of practical sanitation.

In his next letter of 12 October Manson commented as follows on my experiments made to try to infect healthy persons by the bites of mosquitoes and remarked: "Your experiments on mosquito biting are interesting although negative. It may be that the mosquito conveys the parasite in biting but I do not think so—at all events I do not think that it does so directly, for the habit of the mosquito is to bite once only and the normal evolution of the parasite is sure to correspond and to run parallel with the normal habits of the insect. I think you are more likely—assuming that the parasite is conveyed by the bite of the mosquito—to find that it is conveyed by the offspring of the mosquito that has bitten the malariated individual—that it is conveyed by the children and not by the parent seeing that on the flagellum hypothesis it has to evolute in the insect that has bitten and swallowed. You might try feeding mosquitoes on a malariated man, keeping them, rearing their young, and setting these to bite an uninfected subject." As a matter of fact this story of a carrying agent communicating a disease to its progeny and thence to the original host was simply the story of the *Piroplasma bigeminum* of oxen, which is carried by ticks in this manner as previously proved by Smith and Kilborne (page 8). I did not know this at the time, and if Manson knew it he did not mention the fact to me. I proposed to do some work on these lines but am glad that I did not waste time over them.

In March 1896 Manson had developed the whole of his theory in the three Goulstonian Lectures delivered before the College of Physicians in London.[29] He argued the case admirably and reiterated his view that the so-called flagellum is really a flagellated spore which escapes in the stomach cavity of the mosquito in order to infect it. In the second lecture he showed the analogy which exists between his hypothesis and the general principle of metaxeny of parasites, especially in the case of the filaria, partially discovered by him, and then gave his hearers in brief much of what I had written to him, such as the adventures of a flagellum (page 49) and the life history of the mosquito gregarine (page 53). His third lecture was devoted to an exposition of my work during 1895, describing especially the "exflagellation" of crescents in mosquitoes and my conclusions given in my letter of 28 May. And he said that "we may conclude with confidence that Ross has thoroughly proved by direct observation my hypothetical conjectures that the stomach of the mosquito is a suitable medium for the flagellated phase of the *Plasmodium malariae* to develop in." He concluded by countering some possible objections to the theory. The whole lecture should be studied by those who are interested in the development of scientific hypothesis.

But now in his letter of 12 October he sent me something of a bombshell. A Bignami, a Roman physician, had done much admirable work on malaria, especially in conjunction with E Marchiafava, and had considerably extended the work of Laveran and Golgi in detail. His work and that of other Roman writers was brilliant but showed some undue tendency to absorb the credit of previous writers, and he was indeed one of the triumvirate who attempted to pirate my work in 1898. But he now published an article in *Policlinico* of 5 July 1896[30] objecting to Manson's mosquito theory and attempting to substitute one of his own. The objection was based upon what was really a mere speculation—that the flagellate bodies are not living creatures but are dying organisms and that the appearances due to the escaping flagella are really nothing but the dying struggles of these bodies. So far as I can make out this hypothesis had been started some years previously by another member of the triumvirate—namely, B Grassi. The only reason for the speculation was that no one had then succeeded in finding chromatin in the flagella and when Bignami wrote his objections to Manson's theory he did not know that in fact the chromatin had just been found in the flagella by Sakharoff.[31] Indeed Manson had already anticipated this difficulty in his Goulstonian Lectures, but as few people knew the facts and as Bignami was a man of considerable eminence the Indian authorities immediately began to think that Manson and I had been quite mistaken and it was necessary for me to disprove Bignami's contention. Manson had sent me a translation of Bignami's paper[30] and I thought that the paper was trying not only to discredit Manson's hypothesis but also to peg out a claim for a new hypothesis of Bignami's own which, if proved by someone else, would give him and not Manson the credit. This indeed is an old device of Italian literature of this class. An alleged flaw is found in a given theory or investigation, the whole theory or investigation is thus discredited, and the critic then proceeds to repeat it in almost the same terms as now being his own—perhaps with a few alleged experiments in support of it. I was not impressed by the paper because, with Manson, I was already absolutely certain that the flagellate body is not caused by dying struggles but is a living object. But the point was fundamental in our work.

I must have received Bignami's article early in November, and before the end of the month I was able to inform Manson that I had completely disproved his dying-struggle hypothesis. I placed a small lump of vaseline on the patient's finger and pricked his skin through it so as to allow a drop of blood to exude into the vaseline. The whole mass was now removed on to the microscope slide without exposing the blood to the air for a second and was then flattened out and examined. I found that the crescents never underwent the change into spheres and flagellate bodies as described in Chapter 2 but that after 24 hours they all showed signs of disintegration and death. How was this then? Here the crescents died, but they did not show the dying struggles at all. So much for Bignami. On the other hand if the vaseline specimen was opened after only three or four hours, before the crescents had died, and the blood was exposed to the air the crescent-sphere-flagella change went on just as before in blood immediately exposed to the air or contained in the mosquito's stomach. That is, the process was certainly a living process. But at the same time I found the great condition necessary for this metamorphosis, which was abstraction of water from the blood either by exposure to the air or by the stomach of the mosquito. Blood exposed to the air throws out water vapour with great rapidity and it is certain that the mosquito's stomach absorbs water from the contained blood with equal rapidity. If no abstraction of water takes place the crescents do not become transformed. That is, the crescents become transformed only when the conditions which obtain in the mosquito's stomach are present. On 14 November I had already shown that the same transformation goes on in the stomach of leeches—in which of course a similar abstraction of blood occurs—and I asked Manson to confirm these observations and said, "by the way, could you not work the leech in London?" Indeed, all this work could have been done in London and Manson and Manson and Rees confirmed it later.

By 7 December I had repeated these experiments over and over again and finished my paper "On a condition necessary to the transformation of crescents."[32] I had also shown that the longer blood is exposed to the air the more of the crescents become transformed. I received much assistance at that time from Dr Srinivasa Rao. We showed that the flagella generally appear about 11 minutes after the blood is drawn and ascertained many other interesting details, such as the exact manner in which the crescent turns itself into a sphere and then bursts the envelope of the corpuscle containing it. I was rather indignant with Bignami and wrote in the following angry and exaggerated way about him: "He wants to secrete a mosquito theory of his own. He is wild with you. He wants to bite into the heart of your theory, suck its juices, and then bloat and swell into a discoverer—or rather until he is thought to be one.... He is welcome to his epidemiological inductions; they will only lead him face to wall against somebody else's. But he must be dealt with at once with clear distinctions because he is quite capable of spreading his six legs over your work and calling it all his own*; next he will say that he knows about the flagellated spores all along and so on. If you have not squelched him already you ought to do it." Unfortunately, just after I had posted my article to the *British Medical Journal* I found one by Dr Marshall in the *Lancet* of 24 October 1896 in which he showed that flagellation is expedited by *adding* water to the blood. This was really due to a mechanical effect of the water, but my paper was delayed by the necessity of investigating the point thoroughly. I have no space to quote the numerous letters to Manson on these points dated 15 December, 23 December, 27 December (with which we added a note to my article), 11 January 1897, 8 February, 7 March, and 17 March 1898—my last one from Bangalore. My article with appended note appeared in the *British Medical Journal* of 30 January 1897 with a laudatory editorial paragraph;

* Exactly what he tried to do[33] (page 213).

and other notes on the same observations were given before the South Indian branch of the British Medical Association on 29 January 1897 and were published in the *Indian Medical Gazette* a year later. All these researches will interest chiefly biological workers only, who will find full details in the papers mentioned.[32]

After I took charge of the Bowring Civil Hospital in June 1896 I began to study microscopically cases of diarrhoea and dysentery and immediately found numbers of amoebae and flagellates. Of course work on these organisms had to be done during moments snatched from my sanitary labours and my malaria researches and led to nothing remarkable. But I was one of the first in India to deal with these parasites. D D Cunningham in Calcutta had long worked on them but had gone quite wrong and thought that they were innocuous, thus holding back the hand of science for years. I have no space to deal with the matter here but may mention my paper (full of misprints) published in 1897.[34]

During all these researches I had never found that more than 60 % of the crescent-spheres emitted flagella even under the most favourable conditions, the remaining 40 % or more continuing to exist as unchanged crescent-spheres for hours. I could think of no explanation of this, though there was a very simple one—the former were male cells and the latter female cells. The "adventures of a flagellum" which I had seen (page 49) ought to have opened my eyes; and on 16 February 1897, shortly before leaving Bangalore, I observed something which should certainly have revealed the truth to me in a flash. In the blood of a case of quartan (*Plasmodium malariae*) on that date two parasites were lying close together, one emitting a number of struggling "flagella" and the other remaining a perfect sphere with one of the flagella *moving slowly within it*. Here is a copy of the rough drawing on page 87 of my notebook.

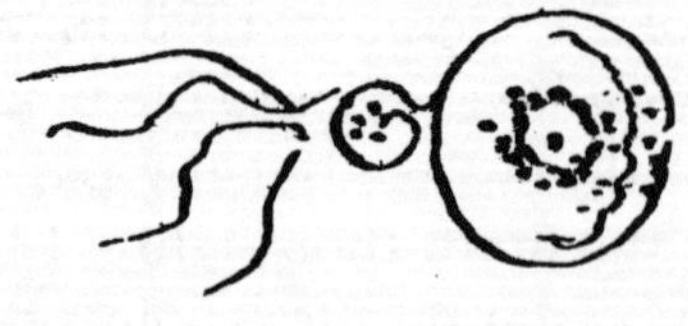

Of course only one sperm enters the female cell, but it did not occur to me that this one had *entered* the sphere—I thought it was *trying to get out*! I was so obsessed by Manson's hypothesis that these sperms were flagellated spores that at that time I never even fancied they could be anything else, though previously I had guessed they might be sperms.

The honour of this discovery therefore fell deservedly to W G MacCallum in America, who actually witnessed some few months later a "flagellum" entering a "crescent-sphere."[35] I have always felt disgraced as a man of science ever since! Simond had previously proved a similar phenomenon in *Coccidium oviforme* of rabbits[36] (pages 130, 141).

Regarding birds' malaria I wrote to Manson on 31 October 1896: "I forgot to tell you that I have tried several pigeons, doves, and paroquets with negative results. This place is 2700 feet above sea level, remember. However, I will look again. I have not been working with animals. I am dying to get away to some regular hotbed of malaria...."

5

The Dappled-winged Mosquito. Sigur Ghat, 1897

In organising the new health department for the Civil and Military Station of Bangalore I had arranged for a health officer, but the salary which could be afforded was not sufficient to provide for an officer of one of the government medical services, such as myself, even if one could be spared. When Surgeon Colonel Dobson took his furlough home in May 1896 he had applied to be promoted from the residency surgeoncy at Bangalore to a better paid one in Rajputana and had hoped that I should be given the post which he was to relinquish so that I might continue to superintend Bangalore sanitation for years. Of course this would have been a good thing for me, but it was not to be because on his return from furlough Dobson found that the Rajputana billet did not suit him and therefore decided to revert to his former appointment—as he was entitled to do. In March 1897 therefore I found myself left with no better employment than my own appointment as medical officer of my regiment, the 19th MI, which was still at Begumpett, Secunderabad. But before rejoining it I took some short leave which was due to me and left Bangalore on 29 March 1897 to join my wife and family at Ootacamund, where they had been for a month in a pretty little house which we had taken there called Blenheim.

At that time the government medical services in India were distributed as follows. The British troops were in the charge of the Army Medical Service, of which there were then, I think, about 400 officers in India who worked chiefly at the big station hospitals, one of which was in each of the garrison towns or stations. The Indian Medical Service (to which I belonged) consisted of about 600 officers and was divided into two branches. The military branch had charge of the Indian troops, each regiment of which possessed its own medical officer; and the civil branch provided the civil medical and sanitary officers throughout the country. We were primarily a military service, the civil surgeons being always subject to recall by the military in case of emergency. The civil surgeons saw most of the medical and surgical practice, especially in the great cities, taught at the medical schools, and had made the service famous by their fine work, especially as regards surgery of the eye, of elephantiasis, and of stone of the bladder. They were generally busy men, but the regimental surgeons, of whom there were often three or four or more in the same station, were seldom occupied for more than an hour or two out of every day—as I have described in the preceding pages. The authorities were obliged to keep up what appeared to be an excessive staff of doctors, partly because of large and sudden demands for frequent military expeditions and partly because of our rules for leave—we were (quite necessarily) allowed one year's furlough to England after five years' service in India as well as two months' "privilege leave" every year and 10 days' or three days' "station leave" when we could occasionally be spared (besides sick leave, of course). All this meant that each regimental medical officer was sometimes in charge of several regiments at once and also that we were often posted about from one station to another at short notice and at great expense to ourselves—since Government frequently refused to pay the full cost on one excuse or another. As regards general administration each presidency possessed its Civil Surgeon General, a senior IMS officer, with his secretary, a more junior one; and also a military Principal Medical Officer with his secretary, both of whom might belong either to the Army or to the Indian Medical Service; while there were also administrative medical officers of numerous districts and commands. Then there were large numbers of assistant surgeons, hospital assistants, compounders, and so on—altogether a very large organisation which, though defective at certain points, did a vast amount of good work. The principal defects were that there was no proper, or indeed scarcely any, provision or encouragement for scientific investigation, no really adequate sanitary service, and no sufficient means for dealing with epidemics. Thus, though plague had broken out for some years in China, almost no precautions had been taken to exclude it from India, except in Madras, so that when it entered in 1896 it fell like an avalanche over the whole country. And in 1897 another demand was made on the medical services by the Tirah (Afridi) campaign in Northern India. These circumstances reduced my chances of being placed on special duty for the investigation of malaria.

In Chapter 2 I mentioned how my employment for such investigation by the Maharaja of Patiala had been refused by Government in 1895; but in Bangalore in 1896 I strove hard to be put on special duty for the purpose after my sanitary work there was concluded. Manson in England pushed hard in the same direction and wrote to many influential people about it—especially to Surgeon General Cleghorn, Director General of the Indian Medical Service. In August 1896 the United Planters' Association held a meeting at Bangalore and on the 14th, after considering papers submitted by me, resolved on the motion of Mr J G Hamilton: "That the secretary be instructed to move the Government of Madras to commence an inquiry into the development of the malarial parasite on somewhat similar lines to the investigation undertaken by Surgeon Major Ross and others.... " In October the Hon Mr Bliss, member of the Madras Executive Council, under whom the civil medical service was placed, came to Bangalore. I called upon him at the residency and he promised to help. The result was that on 30 October the Surgeon General at Madras (civil, Dr Sibthorpe) wrote a handsome letter to the secretary to the Indian Government at Simla asking for me to be specially appointed for the work. While this was being considered at Simla that able officer Surgeon Colonel W G King, sanitary commissioner at Madras, wrote several dispatches urging the same inquiry and pointing out that a place called Pudupett would be suitable for it.

I had now long begun to think that the "brown" and the "brindled" mosquitoes with which only I had worked hitherto (that is, gnats of the genera Culex and Stegomyia, see page 99) could not be the proper malaria-bearing species and on 31 October 1896 wrote to Manson: "I have lately been thinking that the first thing necessary to further investigation is to be sent to a place where I can be pretty sure that the species of mosquito is a malaria-bearing species. I was much struck on reading the Goulstonian Lectures by the supposition that each species of parasite may require a different species of mosquito [this proved to be wrong] and it is indeed otherwise likely that only certain species can harbour the malaria [this proved to be right]. Here for instance, though mosquitoes are plentiful, there is but little malaria. This may obviously be caused by the species of insect, the brown and the brindled, being not the right kind; and if such be the case I cannot expect the flagellated spores to live in their tissues so that I cannot hope to find malaria parasites in their tissues nor to produce malaria by means of them.... What is to be done then? My peons don't seem to be able to get any but the brown or brindled mosquitoes and as these, especially the latter, swarm in every house, while yet there is little malarial fever, I don't suppose that they are malaria-bearing species. The only thing to be done is to go to some very malarial locality, say a malarious village at the foot of hills.... This, accordingly, is what I have asked Government to do with me." And I told him that Mr Bliss was distinctly favourable, detailed my plans for the investigation, and again asked for literature on mosquitoes (none was to be obtained!). I added that I was examining the blood of pigeons, doves, and paroquets for the avian plasmodia—none could be found.

Now, even after five months, no sanction of the investigation had reached me from the Government of India. So, consigning Simla to the plains, I determined to carry it out at my own expense, put my things together, hired extra servants, and asked Dr C McVittie (the military Surgeon General, who was then at Ootacamund) for two months' privilege leave from my regiment at Secunderabad (I had had none since 1893). As everyone knows, Ootacamund is a bit of England placed on the rounded tops of the Nilgiri Hills, about 8000 feet above sea level—open grassy downs with woods of eucalyptus here and there and a lovely climate, without malaria; but the disease abounded in the gullies and trenches which led down from the summits to the surrounding plains. Just when I was ready, however, the Principal Medical Officer at Secunderabad refused my leave owing to scarcity of officers (one of them was then at Ooty *racing*); but the Surgeon General overruled him. I wrote:

BLENHEIM, OOTACAMUND,
13 *April* 1897.

DEAR DR MANSON,

Here I am within a week, I hope, of going into the jungles after the malaria parasite. Dobson relieved me a fortnight ago at Bangalore and I intend now to devote my future to real work. The government investigation has not yet been sanctioned, but I believe it will be sanctioned. I enclose a little fillip I have given them in the *Pioneer* (9 April).* But I have no intention of waiting for them to make up their very sluggish minds and have applied for two months' leave so as to be able to start work at once. The Surgeon General tells me that he will give the leave. My apparatus is ready packed for the jungle work, and as soon as I get my leave definitely I shall commence work at the foot of these

* Merely a short leading article on the necessity for an investigation.

hills at a place where I hear fever is very bad. This place is at the bottom of the Sigur Ghat (*Cañon*), the top of which is only half an hour's run from my house here (on a bicycle). I think, however, that I shall go and live at a dak bungalow lower down the ghat and just above the malaria. However, I intend to make no definite plans until I have looked about a bit. Some weeks will be occupied, I expect, in such "looking about" and I must probably buy tents and get right into the haunts of King Malaria. Tippoogadoo is the name of the place I have heard of. Will write more next mail if things go well. Am dying to be off but can't start till definite orders come.

With kindest regards,

Yours sincerely,

R Ross.

The facts about the sanction for the investigation from Simla were these. On arrival at Ooty I wrote to the secretary to the civil Surgeon General at Madras (Dr Sibthorpe) asking if the sanction had been received. On 22 April he answered: "I am desired to say that no reply has yet been received from the Govt of India on the subject of the malaria investigation." To this letter I appended the note: "I read the reply myself at Govt offices Ooty on the 21st!" Indeed the reply had been sent from Simla on 19 March but had not been communicated to me all this time! This delay was a misfortune for me because on 15 April the secretary of Dr Cleghorn, Director General of the Indian Medical Service at Simla, had wired to me: "Will you be candidate for officiating civil surgeoncy at Akola wire reply." I refused because of the expected malaria investigation—so that I lost the appointment owing to this piece of official incompetence. I found the papers at Ootacamund on the 21st on personal inquiry at the office and still possess all the documents. Doctors are often shocking bunglers at official correspondence. Of course, when offering me the appointment Dr Cleghorn's secretary should have wired to me that the malaria investigation had not been sanctioned. But misfortunes do not come singly, as the following will show.

OOTACAMUND, 28 *April* 1897.

DEAR DR MANSON,

My reconnaissance has had rather an unexpected ending. I went to Kalhutti on Thursday 22nd. On the 23rd I went down to the bottom of the ghat (4 miles) and then 4 miles across the spur of a mountain to another valley where there is Kindersley's coffee estate, Westbury. We had had early tea at 7.30 am, started from Kalhutti at 8 am, and reached the coffee estate at 10.30 or 11.0. Then we had tea which I noticed was coolish, while the milk seemed watered (?). Then we examined a boy with fever (finding malignant tertian) and went to look at the source of drinking water, a puddle fed by a mountain stream or rather a trickle. The puddle was full of frogs and water beetles, etc. Next we walked on the estate, which was under irrigation, the ground and air teaming with life and seething with heat and moisture. We had breakfast at 1.30 (whisky and soda). More coolies examined afterwards, many with spleens; range [?] at 6 pm. On Saturday I examined specimens and on Sunday 25th did the same with several walks in the upper part of the ghat. At 10 pm I was seized with a severe go of fever and had to come back here yesterday.

The fever was bad all night, beginning with a sudden pain in the liver followed by two hours' rigor and then two hours' fever with aching in bones and gradual defervescence. I slept from 4 to 6 am on the 26th and woke feeling all right. I had taken 5 gr quinine on the 22nd, 23rd, and 24th, but 10 gr on Sunday the 25th. As soon as I knew what was wrong I took 20 gr more at once. Hence on Monday morning I found only one small amoeboid body (quite typical and moving) in two excellent specimens. I don't know the species. At 9 am fever began to come on again without rigor and very slightly. I slept till 3 pm, when I woke in much perspiration and have not had fever since. Liver still hurts on a deep breath, but I gave the parasites such a warm reception with quinine that I don't think they liked it. I shall be off down to the ghat again in a few days. Unfortunately had no thermometer with me at Kalhutti, but the fever must have run very high because I felt twitchings all over and was a trifle light-headed I think for a little. Had no phenacetin etc.

Now I slept every night at Kalhutti inside a mosquito net and with closed windows and doors. At Kalhutti there is a planter, Nash, with a few coolies, two of whom had been ill lately with fever. In the dak bungalow where I was the native servant and his wife had both had fever lately. He had a large spleen but no parasites. If front of their hut was a puddle full of mosquito grubs which I am still examining. Neither of my two servants who also slept at Kalhutti have had fever yet. We all drank boiled water and milk religiously.

I must watch developments before judging where I got the fever but think I got it at Westbury, Kindersley's estate at the foot of the ghat, on Friday the 23rd. This gives about 60 hours' incubation period. Anyway the incubation must have been under 72 hours. Kalhutti is 5500 feet up above the sea and Westbury about 3000 feet. 29th. I fear this letter has missed the mail. My case gives useful data to go upon. Assuming the incubation period to have been 48 hours, then with the most rapidly developing species of parasite no more than two generations could have hatched in that time; in other words on the average one parasite admitted on the 23rd could scarcely have become more than 100 parasites on the 25th. Again, on the 25th I suppose that quite one in 10 000 of my corpuscles must have been infected, probably many more. Now I have about 25 000 000 000 000 corpuscles* so that on the 25th I must have had about 2 500 000 000 parasites in my body. Dividing this by 100 we get the number of parasites which I must have taken in on the 23rd—namely, about 25 000 000.

I think you will admit on consideration that this line of reasoning is really quite sound, fantastic as it may seem.† We can roughly estimate the rate at which a quotidian parasite can breed from the number of spores it has and the period of the cycle. All this considered, I think that 25 millions of parasites or spores must have been the least number admitted on the 23rd.

Now on that day I spent nine hours in the malarious region and breathed about 30 inhalations a minute, each inhalation containing about 25 cubic inches of air (vide any physiology textbook). Hence I breathed about 405 000 cubic inches of air during the nine hours. Suppose all the air to have been equally impregnated with malaria germs the 405 000 cubic inches must have contained 25 000 000 germs; or one cubic inch must have contained no less than 62 malaria germs.

This is something unheard of, especially as I was in the malarious region only during the day. The largest number of bacteria found in air is, I believe, something like one bacterium in 10 cubic inches. Here we have 62 sporozoa in one inch! If, however, I contracted the infection while walking in the coffee plantation (one hour) the number of germs there must have been nine times as large—namely, about 558 a cubic inch!

On the other hand if I contracted this infection by drinking the tea,

* A wrong estimate based on old data. Now physiologists would say that I have about 15 000 000 000 000 red corpuscles.

† Manson, who was not mathematical, feared I was still "light-headed" when I wrote all this!

of which I consumed about $1\frac{1}{2}$ pints, we should still get a large number of germs per cubic centimetre but nothing unheard of. Anyway the air or water of the locality must contain large quantities of the material which causes malarial infection. I may add that my case of attack after 48 hours agrees perfectly with report and tradition which speak of numerous persons who have died straight off a day or two after having passed through the lower ghat.

All this appears to me to have a most important bearing on the great problem because it makes us expect to find large numbers of the free form of the germ, whatever it is, in the air and water and ought to facilitate the search. I examined the Westbury water carefully. It did not contain a single mosquito grub, nor did I find one single psorosperm in the mud....

Yours sincerely,
R Ross.

The line of mathematical reasoning, here adopted for the first time, was perfectly correct. It was much amplified later in my *Prevention of Malaria*[3] and led recently to my method of curing parasitic infections by "continuous medication."[37] Certainly I had an attack of malarial fever on Sunday 25 April 1897, but how or where I became infected I do not know for certain. Even if I was infected on the night of 22–23 April the incubation period would have been only 72 hours—an extraordinarily short time—it is generally two or three weeks. But there is a case on record of two or three days' incubation period after the experimental injection of malarious blood very rich in parasites by Bignami (see case 25 in my *Prevention of Malaria*); and if my case was a similar one I should have received an enormous dose of the poison somehow or other on the 22nd–23rd. Of course at that time I had only begun to suspect that infection was carried by the *bites* of mosquitoes (page 72) and still supposed that it lay in drinking water, according to Manson's ideas, so that I thought that I must have drunk some very heavily infected water at Kalhutti. Now we know that infection is carried only by the bites of mosquitoes. Hence if I was infected on the 22nd–23rd I should have been very frequently bitten then. But so far as I knew I was not bitten at all then, and very little later at the foot of the ghat. Was I infected previously in Ootacamund? Just possible but not likely. On jogging my memory, however, I now recollect that I went to look at the Sigur Ghat to see what it was like some time before I first went to Kalhutti on the 22nd—quite possibly about the 14th April. I remember that it was in the evening and that I bicycled some way down the road to Kalhutti, but I cannot remember whether I reached Kalhutti itself on that occasion or not. Certainly there is no note of my having done so either in my notebook (in which other details are carefully recorded) or in my letters to Manson. On the whole I now think it most probable that I was infected by the bite of an infected anopheles on that evening, either at Kalhutti or on the road there.

On 27 April I returned home from Kalhutti a wreck, but I had little more fever, though I found a malaria parasite again in my blood on 29 April. After that I took 10 gr of quinine every day for no less than four months and never had a relapse; but I remained weak and depressed for a long time. In spite of this, however, I worked hard at my specimens and visited the Sigur Ghat again on 5 May and 1 June. On 3 May I wrote Manson a long letter in which I argued that as I had found so few mosquitoes at Westbury and yet had contracted malaria so quickly the malaria parasites in their free stage must be able to multiply enormously in external nature and must be capable only of optional (ie, facultative) parasitism in men and mosquitoes. But this was too hasty a conclusion, for in my next letter I wrote:

OOTACAMUND, 12 *May* 1897.

DEAR DR MANSON,

Another five days in the jungle have reversed the position of affairs in favour of the mosquito theory, but only just as I was beginning to give it up. I started to Kalhutti again on the 5th. On the 6th I went to Sigur, the bottom of the ghat, and spent the whole day there hunting for mosquito pools and examining dew, puddles, etc. Not a mosquito grub to be found. There is a rest house there and in it I found a native with fever. He said he had arrived on 17 April and had been attacked with fever four days afterwards (he may have contracted it on the way). On my intimating that I wanted to examine his blood after breakfast he disappeared. I found, however, a family of nine Kusbahs living all their lives at Sigur in a spot supposed to be absolutely deadly. Not one of them had ever had fever, they said, and certainly none of the seven men and children had spleen. They drank river water. I encamped at this spot during the day on the 6th and 7th May, returning four miles up the ghat to Kalhutti in the evening. I found not a single mosquito grub anywhere but caught a mosquito full of blood in the rest house. This mosquito was small with wings striped *brown* and white.* The Kusbahs (aborigines) informed me that sometimes mosquitoes are so numerous at night that fires are required to keep them off.

On the 8th I descended again and went to Nash's estate two miles out in the plain beyond Sigur. Here 13 out of 16 people had large spleens or fever. They drank out of irrigation streams and lived in the midst of jungle. Even here I could not find a single mosquito pool. The same evening I went on to Westbury, three miles from Nash's plain estate, with intent to live there for a few days (this is where I expect I got my fever at first).

On Sunday 9th I examined water of puddles, mud, everything—not a sign of a mosquito. There was not a mosquito in this bungalow either. I then offered a reward for every mosquito, alive or dead, brought to me and went to bed feeling that mosquitoes could play no essential part in the propagation of malaria.

On the 10th (Monday) I returned to Nash's estate and examined bloods—one case of malignant tertian; looked about a little more and went back to Westbury. Here about 80 % of the people have spleen. Out of 19 Kusbahs I found about half with spleens or fever (women would not be examined). Hence the Kusbahs are by no means immune, though they are partially so compared with other natives on the estates who had come from distant parts. Hence again the fact that the nine Kusbahs at Sigur are free from fever appears to show that that part is free from fever though Nash's estate and Westbury, close by, are so bad. The river at Sigur, from which the nine Kusbahs drink, is, however, a mountain stream running over stones and sand; the streams at Nash's and at Westbury run through rotting vegetation.

After breakfast on the 10th an intelligent native brought me five very small mosquitoes. I jumped with astonishment at the sight of them and told him to take me where he had found them. Instead of taking me to the servants' huts he led me into the neighbouring jungle. It was then midday. He sat down; in one minute four or five mosquitoes had fastened on his black legs and arms, one was on my hand, and several were prospecting my trowsers [*sic*]. I let the one on my hand bite me, which it did in a few seconds, giving a sharp pain like a bee sting. One on the native's legs filled itself in about a minute. These insects abounded in the darkest parts of the jungle which, however, was not a large jungle

* The wings were spotted, not striped. It was the first *Anopheles* I had ever observed!

but rather thin scrub and thorn. I searched everywhere for the grubs but could not find a pool of water anywhere, though it had been raining overnight. Anyway, the adult insects swarmed everywhere in the wood. In the evening we looked again for grubs and at last discovered some in a small pool in a rocky ravine almost entirely sheltered from the sun by thick overhead vegetation and fully half a mile from where we had first found the mosquitoes.

Hence enter *Culex sylvestris* or *nemoris*!*—which I ought to have thought of before. Oddly enough there were none under the tree at Sigur where I encamped. The fact is, they do not frequent single trees but shady glades. They appear to fix on one with voracity morning, noon, evening, or night. They do not enter houses—at least well made ones—though the natives say they come into their huts at night. They breed apparently only in the darkest and most secluded woodland pools in dried-up watercourses and are quite different from the ordinary house mosquito [? in size only].

The adults are very small with brindled bellies and very formidable suctorial apparatus. The grubs are also small, brindled, and with very long air tubes. The adults contain swarms of psorosperms, but in the few which I have yet examined I have not found anything very unusual.... Well then, the *Culex sylvestris* has entirely altered the state of affairs. Where I was just about to give up the theory owing to the absence of mosquitoes I find that mosquitoes are swarming. *If then malaria occupies the mosquito at all it occupies the Culex sylvestris* and I must find it there by hook or by crook.... It looks also as if the bite does it in some way, it appearing to me very questionable whether the forces of dilution in air or water would not reduce the chance of infection almost to an impossibility, even granting that the woods are full of *C sylvestris*. It appears much more likely that infection is brought straight to men (as a rule) by the insect itself....

Yours truly,

R Ross.

Here is an example of the numerous pitfalls which beset the path of the investigator. This swarming *Culex sylvestris* does not carry malaria at all but the single insect "with wings striped brown and white" which I

* Probably a very small variety of *Stegomyia scutellaris* with the same parasites, eggs, and general appearance. I expect that it was breeding in "rot holes" in trees and that the larvae found in the ravine were larvae of some other species. I have forgotten details.

found in the rest house at Sigur was the real culprit! I remember the latter well. Unlike most of the genera Culex and Stegomyia, its wings were *spotted*; and I noticed at once that it sat with its tail sloped at an angle to the wall, while the abdomens of Culex and Stegomyia hang parallel to the wall. It was in fact an anopheline, the malaria-bearing family of mosquito! But this was actually the first time that I had ever seen (or at least noted) one, though I had now been studying mosquitoes and malaria for more than two years. Who would have thought that this "single spy" was the true enemy while the whole "battalions" of the *Culex sylvestris* were innocent? Another four months were, however, fated to pass before I could convict it. On the other hand my conjecture that "the bite does it" was right, but another year was to pass before I could prove it so. The mosquitoes which came into the huts of the natives at night were probably the anopheles and not the culex.

Four more long letters to Manson from Ootacamund dated 16, 24, 31 May and 17 June 1897 were all occupied with minute descriptions of a number of new kinds of parasite which I found in the Sigur mosquitoes—any one of which might have been, for all I knew, the mosquito stage of the malaria parasite. I will not detain the reader with descriptions of these, though they were interesting enough, because some account of them was published in papers to be mentioned presently. In the last of these letters I now gave a list of six kinds of parasite of mosquitoes, all of which except the first were discovered by me—namely:

1. *Filaria bancrofti* (discovered in the mosquito by Manson).
2. A nematode worm.
3. *Gregarina culicis* (probably several species).
4. *Coccidium* (?) *culicis*.
5. *Octosporidium culicis*.
6. Certain flagellate organisms in the stomach and intestine.

I saw also three other classes of object which might have been parasites. On 14 May I gave numbers of the flagellate parasites to one of my servants by the mouth. He had a slight attack of fever on the 20th but no malaria was found in him and I heard subsequently that he was subject to such attacks. Of course he received the usual reward for a "positive result."

My work in the Sigur Ghat proved to my mathematical apprehension that I was "up against" a very difficult problem indeed—an equation containing *two* unknown quantities. There were many species of mosquito and each of these contained many kinds of parasite. How was

I to discover which species of mosquito and which kind of parasite were the right ones? To find one unknown quantity I should be obliged to find the other one simultaneously. There was only one method of solution, that of incessant trial and exclusion. But this meant enormous labour—and I had already spent two years over the quest.

I wrote an account of the work in a paper[38] which I sent to the South Indian branch of the British Medical Association some time before 4 September 1897—when the secretary informed me that it "was considered too long to be read in its entirety before the branch." It contains 13 small pages! Publication was delayed until February 1898, but then it was reproduced in the *Indian Medical Gazette* for May and June 1898 (many printers' errors). I made a mistake in sending so many of my papers to a society which dealt with little else than clinical wonders—such as what I called "wah-wah tumours"—and the proceedings of which were not widely read. This paper was important because of my analysis of the facts hitherto obtained. I inclined to the view that *contact* between men and mosquitoes is the mode of infection; and by contact I meant that the mosquito either inoculates the germ into the wound made by its proboscis or deposits it when defecating on the skin of its victim. On the other hand I admitted that, at least, I had found no further evidence for the mosquito theory in these investigations. Many of the parasites which I saw have since been rediscovered and named by several observers, but I gave a résumé of the subject in the *Journal of Hygiene, Cambridge*,[39] in 1906.

I was now 40 years old and had had 16 years' service; but though I was well known in India, both for my sanitary work at Bangalore and for my researches on malaria, I received no advancement at all for my pains. By a fixed rule an officer passing from one branch of the service to another was obliged to begin at the bottom of the list in the latter branch so that I was practically excluded from entering the civil side of the Madras medical service. Owing to the kind interest of Colonel Robertson, the resident at Bangalore, I was offered an appointment in Rajputana; but this and the appointment at Akola in Berar were by the same rule only very inferior temporary posts and I saw myself condemned for the rest of my service to nothing but regimental work at the lowest salary (for my rank) of about 800 rupees a month. What angered me still more was that not one of my colleagues seemed to take the smallest interest in the malaria work—except Surgeon Colonel King. Even the heads of the service in Madras, Surgeon Generals Sibthorpe and McVittie, did not deign to come and see my specimens at

Ootacamund though I begged them to do so (how little they were interested will be gathered from what follows presently). On the other hand many of the best appointments were filled by men who had really done no special work at all and never intended to do any. When I asked for an extension of leave to continue the malaria work I was refused, though a colleague had been granted six months' leave there for racing. In short, my prospects were not good enough and I determined to retire on my first pension, which would be due to me in a year. But first I wished to make one more desperate effort to solve the Great Problem and therefore wrote on 12 and 20 June to Manson describing my position and begging him to try to have me placed on one year's special duty for this almost forlorn hope before I left the service. I was much discouraged and far from well.

So far as I remember I wrote no verses during my "holidays" except the sections of *In Exile* labelled "Truth-service," "Self-service," and "Wraths"—bitter, perhaps, but justified. Somewhere else, however, and I think previously, those words which come near the end of the poem had been composed:

By that we have we lose;
By what we have not, get;
And where we cannot choose
The crown of life is set.

So it was indeed. I could not choose but to return to Secunderabad; and there, two months later, the Great Problem was to be solved!

6

The Discovery. Secunderabad, 1897

Leaving my wife and family at Ootacamund (where the latter all caught whooping cough a little later), I started on the 16th, spent the 17th at Bangalore, and reached Secunderabad at 6 pm on 18 June 1897.* There I rejoined my regiment, the 19th Madras Infantry, at Begumpett Lines, situated near the outflow of the Husein Saugar Lake, and lived in a good bungalow with Lieut Heffernan, the adjutant, and another officer. My pay was the usual 800 rupees a month but was reduced by quite 100 rupees a month by regimental expenses as I was the next senior officer to the commandant; so that I drew only about half the salary I had in Bangalore. The weather was pleasant when I arrived, but soon, instead of the cooling monsoon rains which ought to have fallen by that date, there came only a raging hot wind with clouds of dust which shrivelled us up. The life itself was pleasant and all the officers, Major Packenham, Captain Harding, Lieut Knox, and others, and the ladies of some of them, were very nice people. In the evenings we played cricket in the maidan opposite the mess and then went to the club; and instead of a pony and trap I used my excellent bicycle. All my doings during this eventful time are recorded in almost daily letters to my wife, besides numerous letters to Manson.

My first experience was far from pleasant. There was a guest night dinner at mess on 25 June and we enjoyed a delicious ice cream pudding. The agony commenced a little after midnight. All five of us suffered—and so, we were glad to hear, did some of the servants (whose caste prejudices forbade them to touch our food!). Cholera was in the

* Wrongly put July 1897 in my Nobel Lecture—which was written chiefly from memory and might have been more exact in some small details.

station and Major Fawcett, the staff surgeon, said next day that he considered we had got that disease—but as bacteriology had scarcely reached India yet (17 years after the discovery of the cause of cholera) we did not know for certain. The same cream had been provided for another dinner party on that night and the wife of our brave general, General Tucker, afterwards of South African fame, was attacked at the same time and died a week later. Mine was the most serius case of our batch and I kept myself alive by drinking cup after cup of scalding hot tea without sugar or milk, swallowing another cupful as soon as a previous one had been rejected. I had thought out and tried to use this line of treatment during the cholera outbreaks in Bangalore in 1896—the object of it being to maintain the water content and the pressure of the blood on the lines of the intravenous injection of salt solution so successfully employed later by Sir Leonard Rogers. Next day Dr Fawcett looked very grave and I felt intensely cold for some days afterwards, as I did in a previous similar attack in Madras.

My next adventure was more amusing. As soon as he heard that I had arrived in Secunderabad Surgeon Colonel Lawrie (page 60) challenged me, not to a duel but to a mortal logomachy over the malaria parasite. I was to bring my own cases to Chudderghat (some 11 miles from Secunderabad) and to demonstrate the plasmodium before him and the full faculties and students of the Nizam's medical school in formal debate assembled. Well, I found a good case in my hospital and on 11 July at 8 am the man's blood was swarming with the youngest stages of *Plasmodium falciparum*. I put him into a bullock cart with a hospital assistant and a handsome tip, dispatched him to Chudderghat, wired to Lawrie, and followed after breakfast. We arrived about noon. Lawrie came into the arena (a lecture room) with about 30 native professors and students, all looking very serious. Not a single parasite could I now find in the patient's blood! Of course, as the Italians had shown, the young stages of this species retire into the inner organs some few hours after their first appearance, but though I was familiar with this phenomenon I did not expect the disappearance to be so speedy. It was not only speedy but complete! Lawrie was very polite but some of the students tittered. I was absolutely routed and did not even dare to describe my defeat to Manson. Not as with prophets do the miracles of the scientist always succeed. It was like St Paul before Agrippa, but I did not almost convert Lawrie to "Laveranity." He was indeed one of the many good surgeons and passable doctors who have no clear conception of what science means.

There was next to no official work to do in the regiment and therefore a junior Indian officer of the IMS named Dr Kanga was appointed to help me to do it. There were numerous doctors in the station and I offered the Principal Medical Officer, Surgeon Colonel N B Major, AMS, to instruct as many of his officers as he pleased in the mysteries of the plasmodium. I believe he published a notice to this effect in station orders, but, so far as I remember, only two officers came to me at that time, Surgeon Captain C A Johnston, IMS, and a Dr Foulkes, who worked with me for some weeks in July—they and Dr Sturmer of Madras being, I think, the only government officers who did so. The PMO himself was not interested. Yet malaria was the commonest disease in the country and was perhaps the principal cause of expense during military expeditions. In fact few men in the whole of India were then doing sound work on the subject. One very good article, "The malaria parasites at Lahore" by C H Murray, appeared in the *Scientific Memoirs by Medical Officers in India* for 1897, but it did not touch the mosquito theory and I did not see it till much later.

On arrival at Secunderabad I indited a report (dated 12 July) on my work in the Sigur Ghat for the Director General of our service and on 20 July his secretary, Surgeon Captain Leslie, wrote to me from Simla that Surgeon General Cleghorn "considers the paper original and highly interesting, and that, when the state of the service permits, he will endeavour to provide you with more favourable opportunities for carrying on your researches than are at present possessed by you." This gave me great encouragement; and in fact on 25 June Dr Leslie had wired me: "Do you wish to become a candidate for a civil surgeoncy in the Central Provinces?" and then on 27 June had wired again: "You will probably get an appointment under the Foreign Office soon but cannot say when." I replied that I left the matter in the Director General's hands and I felt somewhat reassured but also—well, the reader shall see!

On 27 July I received two letters from Manson in reply to mine from Ootacamund complaining of my prospects. He had taken instant action and sent me a copy of an admirable letter which he had written to Sir Charles Crosthwaite of the India Office in London urging that my malaria work should be encouraged and that I should not be driven to take my pension (which would be due to me on 23 June 1898). I cannot forbear quoting the following fine and exact passage: "To our national shame be it said that few, very few of the wonderful advances in the science of the healing art which have signalised recent years have been made by our countrymen. This is particularly apparent in the matter of tropical diseases in which we should, in virtue of our exceptional opportunities, be *facile princeps*. But even in tropical diseases Frenchmen, Italians, Germans, Americans, and even Japanese are shooting ahead of us. We have to get a Koch to find for us the cholera germ and a Haffkine to protect us from it, a Laveran to teach us what malaria is, a Kitasato to show us the germ of plague, and a Yersin or a Haffkine to cure us of its effects.... But in this matter of malaria here is a chance for an Englishman to rehabilitate our national character and to point out to the rest of the world how to deal with the most important disease in the world—malaria." Manson hoped even to reach those Awful Presences the Secretary of State and the Viceroy—then Lord George Hamilton and Lord Elgin; and he succeeded. He added that there was no one so competent in India for the proposed malaria investigation as myself and that it would take years of toil for anyone else to work up to the point reached by me. As a matter of fact, no one else was working at the mosquito theory at all. Out of the thousand million people in the world I believe I was the only one who had been so foolish as to waste leisure, money, and advancement on such a wild goose chase. The Italians, French, and Americans were doing nothing at all and even Manson himself did not try English mosquitoes but left the inquiry to me.

But now the predestined day was approaching and the Power that "shapes our ends, rough-hew them as we may" took the matter out of the hands of the incompetents. I will try to reconstruct the events as exactly as I can out of my notebooks, letters, and memories. On arrival at Secunderabad after the severe labour in Ootacamund I felt my first violent reaction against the microscope and could scarcely bring myself to look through mine for a month. The Great Monsoon seemed to have failed. The hot blast which, instead of it, struck us in June was followed by a suffocating stillness and the sky was filled with a haze of dust through which the sun glared like a foiled enchanter.

The desert is white with heat
Intol'rable, and the smoke of the burning sand
Fills all the air....
What cast of thin vapour covers the flaming sky
And why on his throne so sickly pale the Sun
Erstwhile of the brazen empyrean lord?
What ails him who harms us that his lips are pale—
Pale, and his javelins wreak his wrath no more;
And while his withering lips and his spectral hair
So scatter'd with fear?*

* From my "Indian Shepherds."[40]

Well do I remember those awful days—and nights. I spent the time doing almost nothing but (I believe) writing—or rather moulding in the mind—the stanzas of *In Exile*, Part VII[41]:

What ails the solitude?
  Is this the Judgement Day?
The sky is red as blood;
  The very rocks decay

And crack and crumble, and
  There is a flame of wind
Wherewith the burning sand
  Is ever mass'd and thin'd.
. . . . .

The world is white with heat;
  The world is rent and riven;
The world and heavens meet;
  The lost stars cry in heav'n.

I do not boast my premonitions because they seldom come true! But at that time I was certainly much exalted in spirit and said to myself: "One more effort and the thing will be done." I remember especially a dreadful evening when I climbed one of the heaps of great boulders piled upon each other which dot the plain outside the station and saw the vulture and the dead jackal (mentioned in the poem) below. Then it was that the thought struck me: Why not see whether mosquitoes fed on malaria blood as before contain any of the mosquito parasites which I had found in the Sigur Ghat? I was at full work again on 21 July 1897 on the last lap.

The position of the investigation was now as follows: Manson's theory consisted of two parts. The first part was that the crescent-sphere-flagella metamorphosis was intended to occur in the mosquito's stomach. This was a great and ineluctable induction which I had verified two years previously in this very place. But I had got no further because the second part of his theory—that the liberated "flagella" live in the insect's tissues, from which they enter drinking water—was not nearly so strong, indeed not true. They might, for example, be voided at once by the mosquito on to its victim's skin or even upon the ground of malarious places. In fact they do none of these things but enter and fertilise the female plasmodia. Manson, even in his last letters, kept advising me to "follow the flagellum," but if I had done so I would merely have returned to the point whence I started. My plan now was simply that of 1895, to examine each "malariated mosquito" for any parasites which it might contain but to do so much more thoroughly than before and in the light of my Sigur experiences.

Then the *species* of mosquito had to be considered. In spite of all efforts I had been able to obtain no useful literature on mosquitoes (Culicidae) and knew no one whom I should address on the subject; and though I had sent many of the insects to Manson, none of them had been zoologically classified except one, which he wrongly thought was *Culex pipiens*. Hence, pending further information, I had been obliged ever since 1895 to use a rough classification of my own. I recognised two main groups among the more common moqitoes with which I had been working—namely:

(A) *Grey or barred-back mosquitoes* (mostly *Culex fatigans* Wied), which bit at night, had plain wings, and sat on a wall with tail sloped towards it. Their eggs were shaped like rifle cartridges and were laid packed side by side in clusters, and their larvae had a long breathing tube and floated head downwards. Very like the common English gnat called *Culex pipiens*.

(B) *Brindled mosquitoes* (mostly *Stegomyia fasciata* Fabr and *Stegomyia scutellaris* Walker), which bit in the daytime, had plain wings, and sat like A. But their eggs were oval and laid singly and their larvae had a short breathing tube, but also floated head downwards like those of A.

But in the Sigur Ghat I had found (page 88) a single mosquito of quite another type which I noted, then and in 1898, to have the following characters:

(C) *Dappled-winged mosquitoes* (Subfamily Anophelina), which bite at night, have spotted wings, and sit on a wall with tail sloped away from it. Their eggs are boat-shaped, laid singly, and often lie together touching each other end to end so as to form equilateral triangles. Their larvae have no breathing tube and float flat on the surface of the water like sticks.

The main zoological character which is taken to distinguish groups A and B (Subfamily Culicina) from group C (the Anophelina) is that in the former the females have short palpi and in the latter have long ones. The bodies of the culicines are also much less graceful than those of the anophelines, which seem to be more suitable for longer flight.

To resume, then. About the middle of July I hired three natives to look far and wide for mosquitoes, adults and larvae, but for a month they brought me nothing but groups A and B. On 21 July a case with fairly numerous crescents come to hospital and as I had long thought that these groups were not connected with malaria I now determined to try them again with the most scrupulous care. On 27 July I wrote to Manson: "The experience gained in the Sigur Ghat has given me confidence and knowledge.... I am of course sticking to the flagellulae again but on a slightly modified principle. Owing to their extreme delicacy I doubt whether they can be directly followed into the insect's tissues, but this difficulty can be avoided in a simple manner. The question I have set myself to answer, and which I now feel myself able to tackle, is: 'Do healthy mosquitoes, fed on malarial blood, contain any parasite which similar mosquitoes fed on normal blood do not contain?'... I keep mosquitoes, after feeding on crescents, for one, two, three... days and then examine so as to allow the flagellulae time, by supposition, to mature into full grown mosquito parasites.... Suspicious bodies being noted, I have only to compare with control insects.... Another question, however, must be held in mind: 'Do mosquitoes fed on malarial blood *evacuate* any protozoa not evacuated under similar circumstances by mosquitoes fed on healthy blood?' It may take weeks or years to obtain answers to these questions.... I dissect each malariated mosquito with the utmost care and then search every micron [μm] of it (a micron is one thousandth part of a millimetre) with an oil-immersion. Each mosquito takes about two hours' work.... The things are there and must be found! It is simply a matter of hard work." On 4 August I wrote: "No parasite has been found.... I shall not miss a cytozoon, a spore, an amoeba, or a flagellum, believe me," and on 11 August: "No definite results; and I expect that I must soon state: (*a*) that the brindled species I have been examining are not the hosts of the flagellulae of crescents or spring tertian, or (*b*) the flagellulae develop in them into something very delicate, or very small, or very rare, or almost indistinguishable from normal cells or nuclei."

The monsoon broke a month later in the evening after an awful day, 16 July; and I described the Great Cloud near the end of *In Exile*:

Art thou an Angel—speak,
  Stupendous Cloud that comest?
What wrath on whom to wreak?
  Redeemest thou, or doomest?

But the weather became very hot again in August. At first I toiled comfortably, but as failure followed failure I became exasperated and worked till I could hardly see my way home late in the afternoons. Well do I remember that dark, hot little office in the hospital at Begumpett with the necessary gleam of light coming in from under the eaves of the veranda. I did not allow the punka to be used because it blew about my dissected mosquitoes, which were partly examined without a cover glass, and the result was that swarms of flies and of "eye flies"—minute little insects which try to get into one's ears and eyelids—tormented me at their pleasure, while an occasional stegomyia revenged herself on me for the death of her friends. The screws of my microscope were rusted with sweat from my forehead and hands and its last remaining eyepiece was cracked!

By 15 August 31 mosquitoes of types A and B, all bred from the larva and fed on malarial patients, had been scrupulously examined, not counting numerous unfed mosquitoes, bad dissections, partial dissections, and other studies, including a rat swarming with trypanosomes (thus I had once watched four "flagella" simultaneously attacking a lymphocyte—page 144). On the previous day I had written to my wife: "I have failed in finding parasites in mosquitoes fed on malaria patients, but perhaps am not using the proper kind of mosquito." Now, as if in answer, some Angel of Fate must have met one of my three "mosquito men" in his leisurely perambulations and must have put into his hand a bottle of mosquito larvae, some of which I saw at once were of a type different from the usual culex and stegomyia larvae. Next morning, the 16 August, when I went again to hospital after breakfast the hospital assistant (I regret I have forgotten his name) pointed out a small mosquito seated on the wall with its tail *sticking outwards*. I caught it by my method of placing the mouth of a bottle *slowly* over it—if one jabs the bottle quickly the insect always escapes sideways—and killed it with tobacco smoke. It had spots on the wings* and was evidently like the insect which I had found in the rest house at Sigur (page 88) and is described in my notebook as "a brown mosquito, not brindled, with three black bars on wings caught in ward." I dissected it at once and found nothing unusual; but while I was doing so—I remember the details well—the worthy hospital assistant ran in to say that there were a number of mosquitoes of the same class which had hatched out in the bottle that my men had brought me yesterday. Sure enough there they were: about a dozen big brown fellows, with fine tapered bodies and spotted wings,† hungrily trying to escape through the gauze covering of the flask which the Angel of Fate had given to my humbler retainer—dappled-winged mosquitoes, type C, the first I had ever found in Secunderabad but larger than the one I had just caught on the wall.

* Probably *Anopheles culicifacies*.

† Probably *Anopheles stephensi*.

Immediately my patient, Husein Khan, a man with fairly numerous crescents (and also filariae) was stripped and put on the bed under the mosquito net. This was at 12.25 pm by my notebook; and in five minutes 10 of the new mosquitoes had gorged themselves on him and were caught by the hospital assistant, each in its separate test tube with a drop of water to drink and a loose lump of cotton wool to prevent escape—Husein Khan received one anna for each. At 12.40 and 12.50 pm I dissected two of the insects at once in order to watch the crescent-sphere-flagella metamorphosis in them. I saw little of it in them, but found a filaria of 200 to 250 μm in length, and with a sheath, in one of them. That evening I wrote to my wife: "I have found another kind of mosquito with which I am now experimenting and hope for more satisfactory results with it."

Next day, 17 August, two of my new beauties (*A stephensi*) were dead, but I dissected two of the survivors, mosquitoes 32 and 33. They are described in my notebook as "large, legs, proboscis, and anterior border of wings spotted dark brown and white—brown spots on tail joint of body. Back of abdomen and thorax light brown, belly dark brown. Wings nearly white." I was rather excited over the dissections, spoiled them, and found nothing; and spent the rest of the day examining a flea taken from the rat with trypanosomes.

On the 18th no notes were made in my book, but I wrote to Manson: "I am now beginning on a large, voracious, light brown species with brindled legs and proboscis and thin black bars on the wings—like one of the Sigur species—a kind which I have obtained here with some difficulty." In fact, though I told my mosquito men to remember where exactly they obtained their samples, the fellow who brought me the anopheles could not recollect the point and could get me no more on 16 and 17 August.

On the 19th there were some more anopheles (*A stephensi*) recently hatched out in the original bottle,* and I fed and dissected two of these at once to watch the crescent-sphere-flagella metamorphosis. Nothing else was found and the metamorphosis occurred in mosquito 34 just as it did in stegomyia and culex. But I noted the peculiar eggs of the new type and described them as "large and black, boat-shaped with central spines." Here is the rough drawing of one from my notebook, page 106:

* In my Nobel Lecture these two are confused with the insects fed on the 16th. I must have misunderstood my laboratory notes—hasty scrawls. The present account is correct.

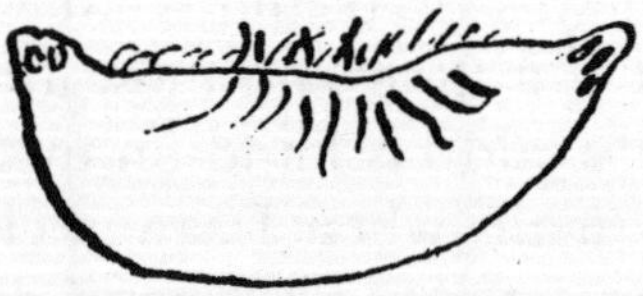

Egg of dappled-winged mosquito.

After this I killed the third "malariated" anopheles of 16 August (mosquito 35) and on dissecting it found some "peculiar vacuolated cells in stomach about 10 μm in diameter." But I added no further note about these cells and do not remember to have thought much about them at the time. This was a mosquito of the third day after feeding so that the blood in its stomach had been evacuated; but the dissection was a poor one and I possessed three more insects of the same batch which I proposed to examine on the morrow—in order to allow the supposed parasites in them to grow as large and as visible as possible. At that time I still credited Manson's idea that mosquitoes feed only once and then die after laying their eggs on the water. I was rather disheartened at my results with the new species but hoped for better things next day.

The 20 August 1897—the anniversary of which I always call Mosquito Day—was, I think, a cloudy, dull, hot day. I went to hospital at 7 am, examined my patients, and attended to official correspondence but was much annoyed because my men had failed to bring any more larvae of the dappled-winged mosquitoes and still more because one of my three remaining anopheles had died during the night and had swelled up with decay. After a hurried breakfast at the mess I returned to dissect the cadaver (mosquito 36) but found nothing new in it. I then examined a small stegomyia which happened to have been fed on Husein Khan on the same day (the 16th)—mosquito 37—which was also negative of course. At about 1 pm I determined to sacrifice the seventh anopheles (*A stephensi*) of the batch fed on the 16th, mosquito 38, although my eyesight was already fatigued. Only one more of the batch remained.

The dissection was excellent and I went carefully through the tissues, now so familiar to me, searching every micron with the same passion and care as one would search some vast ruined palace for a little hidden treasure. Nothing. No, these new mosquitoes also were going to be a failure: there was something wrong with the theory. But the stomach tissue still remained to be examined—lying there empty and flaccid before me on the glass slide, a great white expanse of cells like a large courtyard of flagstones, each one of which must be scrutinised—half an hour's labour at least. I was tired and what was the use? I must have examined the stomachs of a thousand mosquitoes by this time. But the Angel of Fate fortunately laid his hand on my head and I had scarcely commenced the search again when I saw a clear and almost perfectly circular outline before me of about 12 μm in diameter. The outline was much too sharp, the cell too small to be an ordinary stomach cell of a mosquito. I looked a little further. Here was another, and another exactly similar cell.

The afternoon was very hot and overcast and I remember opening the diaphragm of the substage condenser of the microscope to admit more light and then changing the focus. *In each of these cells there was a cluster of small granules, black as jet* and exactly like the black pigment granules of the plasmodium crescents. As with that pigment, the granules numbered about 12 to 16 in each cell and became blacker and more visible when more light was admitted through the diaphragm. I laughed and shouted for the hospital assistant—he was away having his siesta. "No, no," I said, "Dame Nature, you are a sorceress, but you don't trick me so easily. The malarial pigment cannot get into the walls of the mosquito's stomach; the flagella have no pigment; you are playing another trick upon me!" I counted 12 of the cells, all of the same size and appearance and all containing exactly the same granules. Then I made rough drawings of nine of the cells on page 107 of my notebook, scribbled my notes, sealed my specimen, went home to tea (about 3 pm), and slept solidly for an hour. Here is a facsimile of page 107, exactly as written on that day (Plate IV).

When I awoke with mind refreshed my first thought was: Eureka! The problem is solved! I seemed to have found in my sleep an explanation of the pigment. The flagellated spores grow in the gastric cells of the dappled-winged mosquitoes just as the young plasmodia grow in the human blood cells, and as they grow they absorb haemoglobin from the blood in the mosquito's stomach just as the young plasmodia absorb it from the blood cell (the "pigment" is of course nothing but altered haemoglobin). I was wrong: my cells were in fact the *female crescents themselves* (Plate I, figs 22, 23) which had been fertilised by the sperms of the male crescents (which we had called flagellated spores) and were now beginning to grow (Plate I, figs 24, 25), *still containing their original pigment*, in the gastric cells of the anopheles. Scientifically they are called zygotes. But any explanation was enough at the time and I wrote that evening to my wife: "I have seen something very suspicious in my mosquitoes today and hope it may lead to something." Then I added: "Lately I have been putting together those rhymes I used to make on 'exile'—you remember. I think I will write them out fair..." But another consideration struck me. If these cells were the parasites they should *grow in size* in the last remaining mosquito during the night; and I spent that night in an agony lest my sole surviving friend should perish and go bad before morning!

Next day I went to hospital intensely excited. The last survivor of the batch fed on the 16th, mosquito 39, was alive. After looking through yesterday's specimen I slew and dissected it with a shaking hand. *There were the cells again*, 21 of them, just as before, *only now much larger*! Mosquito 38, the seventh of the batch fed on the 16th, was killed on the fourth day afterwards—that is, on the 20th. This one was killed on the 21st, the fifth day after feeding, and the cells had grown during the extra day. The cells were therefore parasites and, as they contained the characteristic malarial pigment, were almost certainly the malaria parasites growing in the mosquito's tissues.

The thing was really done. As I said on page 91, we had to discover two unknown quantities simultaneously—the kind of mosquito which carries the parasite and the form and position of the parasite within it. We could not find the first without knowing the second nor the second without knowing the first. By an extremely lucky observation I had now discovered both the unknown quantities at the same moment. The mosquito was the anopheles and the parasite lives in or on its gastric wall and can be recognised at once by the characteristic pigment. All the work on the subject which has been done since then by me and others during the last 25 years has been mere child's play which anyone could do after the clue was once obtained.

That evening I wrote to my wife: "I have seen something very promising indeed in my new mosquitoes," and I scribbled the following unfinished verses in one of my *In Exile* notebooks in pencil:

This day designing God
Hath put into my hand
A wondrous thing. And God
Be praised. At His command,

I have found thy secret deeds
Oh million-murdering Death.

I know that this little thing
A million men will save—
Oh death where is thy sting?
Thy victory oh grave?

On the 22nd I wrote to my wife, after mentioning the poem again: "I really think I had done the mosquito theory at all [? last], having found something in mosquitoes fed on malaria patients exactly like the malaria parasite." Then, or a few days later, I wrote the following amended verses on a separate slip of paper:

This day relenting God
Hath placed within my hand
A wondrous thing; and God
Be praised. At His command,

Seeking His secret deeds
With tears and toiling breath,
I find thy cunning seeds,
O million-murdering Death.

I know this little thing
A myriad men will save.
O Death, where is thy sting?
Thy victory, O Grave?

About the same time the two subsequent sonnetelles of *In Exile* were added—also on separate slips for tentative arrangements; and I did not like to change them further when they were published 13 years later. The three final sonnetelles of *In Exile* had been written previously and the poem was now finished, though I did not know it then.

Reviewing this work after nearly a quarter a century I still think that no other method but mine would have solved the problem. There was no evidence to incriminate the anopheles by themselves: they are seldom more numerous than other kinds of mosquito, even in the most malarious areas; they often abound only for brief periods; frequently they enter houses only during the night and leave again at daybreak; and by no means all species even of the anophelines carry malaria. It would therefore have been impossible to obtain any genuine statistical evidence of their guilt. So also regarding the parasites in the mosquitoes; there was absolutely no clue to indicate a priori their form and position in the insects. There was only one sound method of procedure—the old one of incessant "trial and failure." But this meant an enormous amount of work. It was that extra half hour's work on 20 August which gave the clue, but even then the success was a miracle of luck. I think that but for this the problem would not have been solved today or perhaps even centuries hence.

After my work was published near the end of the year a number of

Plates

PLATE I

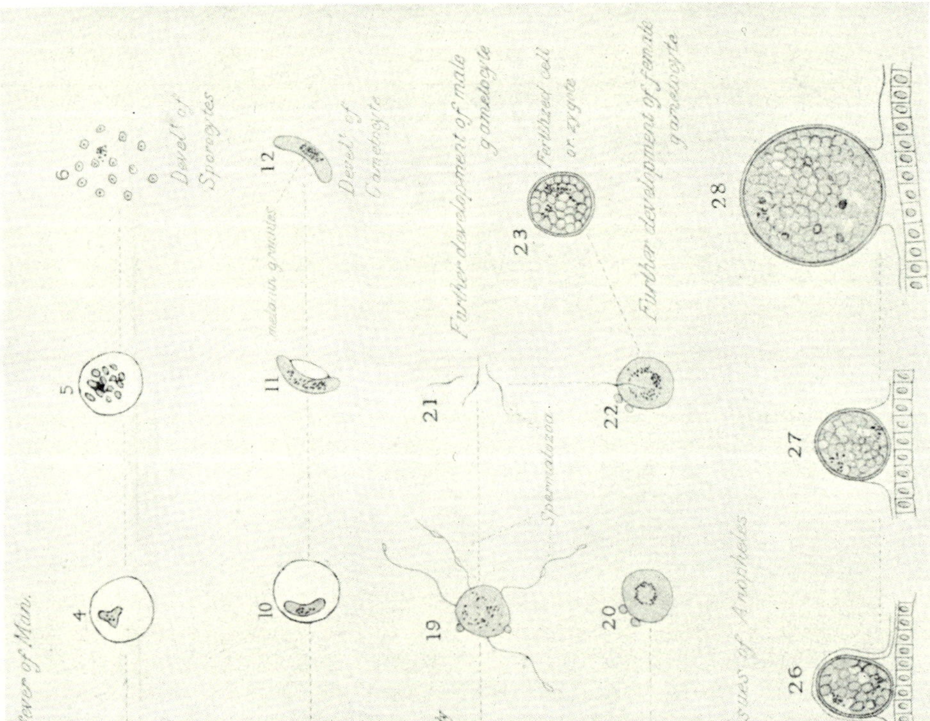

Life history of Plasmodia.

Description of Plate I—Life history of the Plasmodia.

(From article by R Ross and R Fielding-Ould, *Journ Micros Science*, 1900)

FIGS 1–6—Asexual life of *Plasmodium falciparum* (or *Hæmomenas præcox*) in human blood.

FIG 1—Spore

FIG 2—Spore in red corpuscles.

FIGS 3, 4—Growth of young parasite in red corpuscle.

FIG 5—Parasite matures and forms spores.

FIG 6—Corpuscle bursts and spores are scattered in the blood-fluid.

FIGS 7–12—Sexual life of *P falciparum* in human blood.

FIG 7—Spore.

FIGS 8–10—Growth of young parasite in red corpuscle.

FIGS 11, 12—Mature sexual parasites (called crescents).

FIGS 13–23—Changes of the sexual forms of *P falciparum* in the blood contained in stomach cavity of Anopheles.

FIGS 13, 15, 17—The male crescent swells up and becomes round.

FIG 19—It emits sperms (formerly called flagella).

FIG 21—Free sperms.

FIGS 14, 16, 18, 20—The female crescent becomes round.

FIG 22—A sperm enters the female cell.

FIG 23—The fertilised female cell, or zygote.

FIGS 24–38—Diagrams of the general development of the plasmodia in the tissues of mosquitoes.

FIGS 24, 25—The zygote breaking through stomach wall of mosquito.

FIGS 26–28—Zygote attached to outer coat of stomach and growing in size.

PLATE I (*continued*).

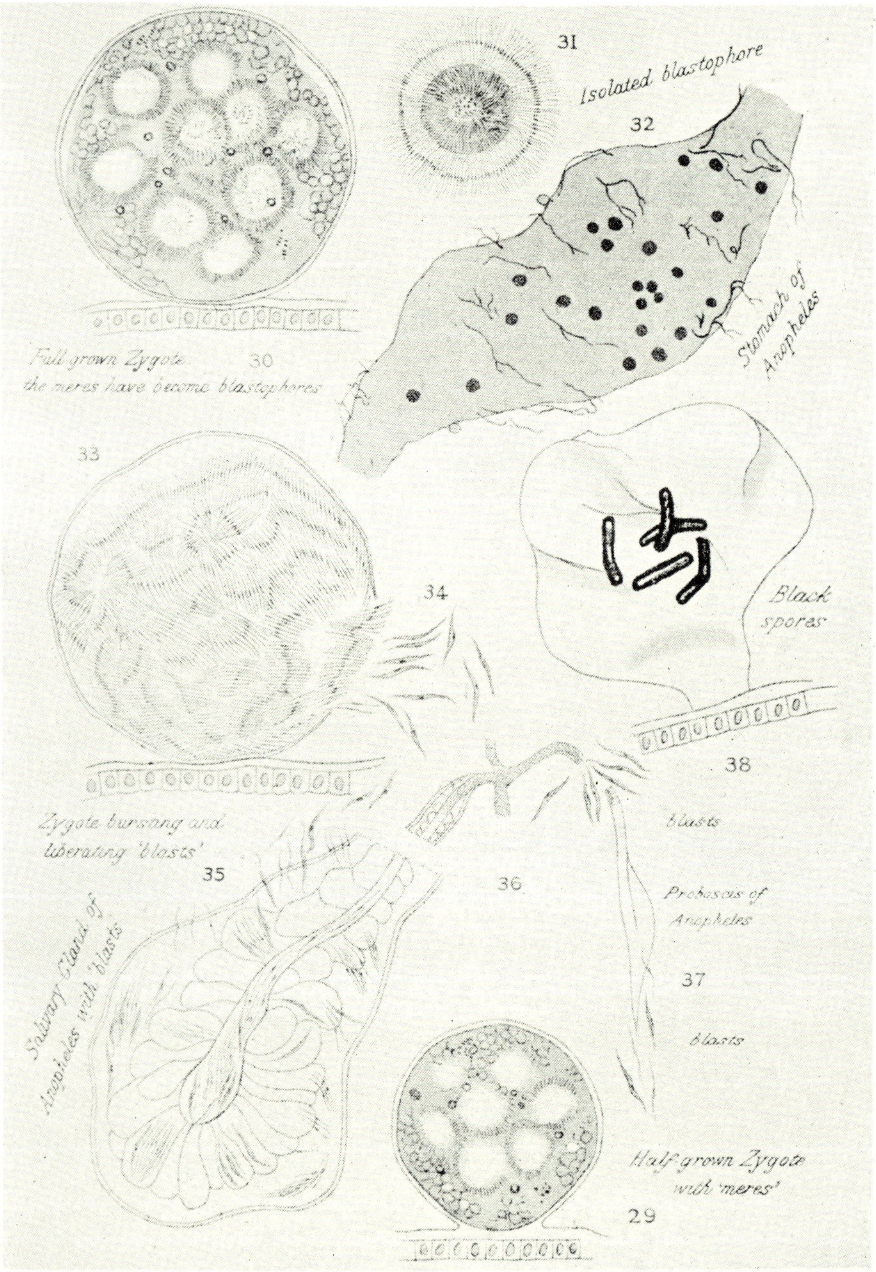

Life history of Plasmodia (*continued*).

FIG 29—Zygote attached to outer coat of stomach and growing in size.

FIG 30—Mature zygote (oocyst) containing blastophores.

FIG 31—A single blastophore with blasts attached by their ends to a central sphere.

FIG 32—Stomach of mosquito with mature zygotes attached (low magnification).

FIG 33—The central sphere of the blastophore is absorbed, leaving the mature zygote packed full of blasts.

FIG 34—The zygote ruptures and the blasts (protospores, sporozoites) escape into the mosquito's blood.

FIG 35—The blasts enter the mosquito's salivary gland.

FIGS 36, 37—They pass up the ducts of the gland and escape by the central stabling lancet in the mosquito's proboscis into blood again.

FIG 38—The capsule of an empty zygote containing some "black spores."

PLATE II

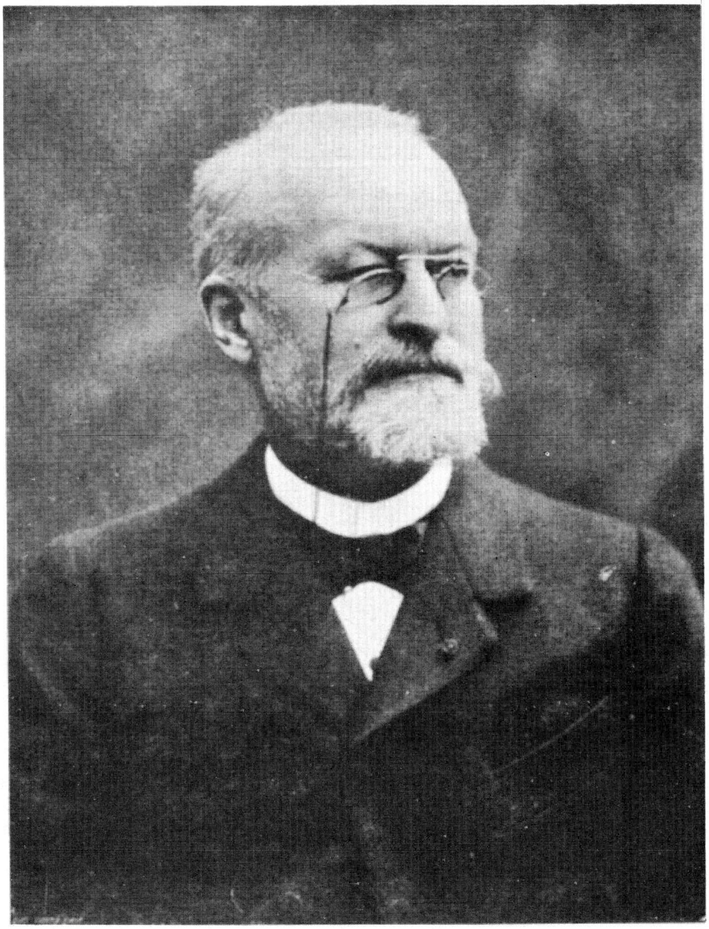

Charles Louis Alphonse Laveran.

PLATE III

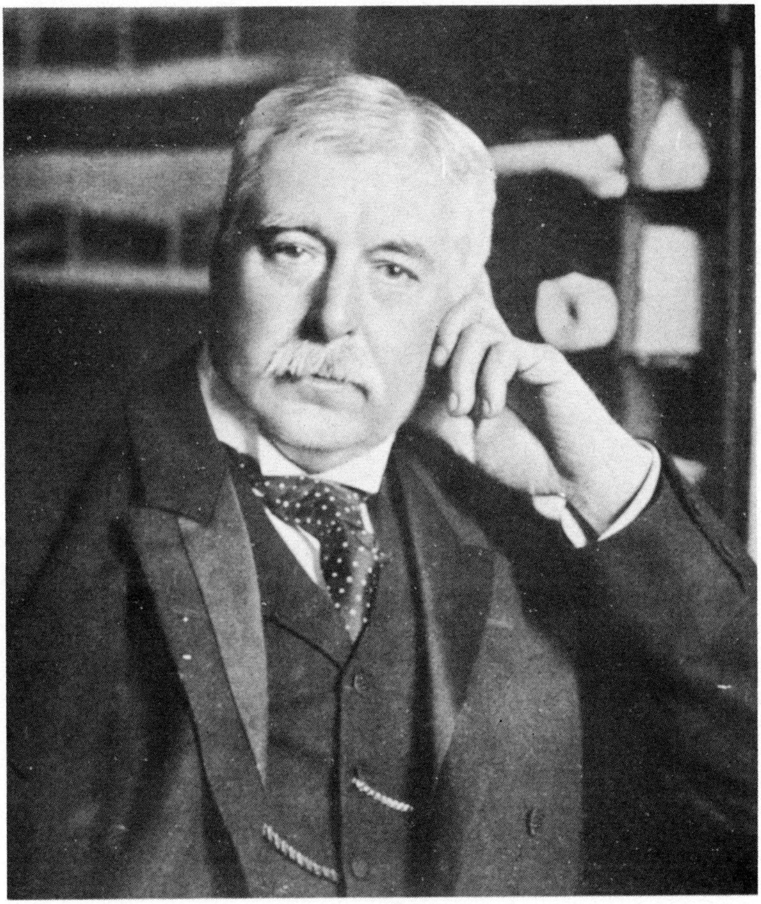

Patrick Manson.

PLATE IV

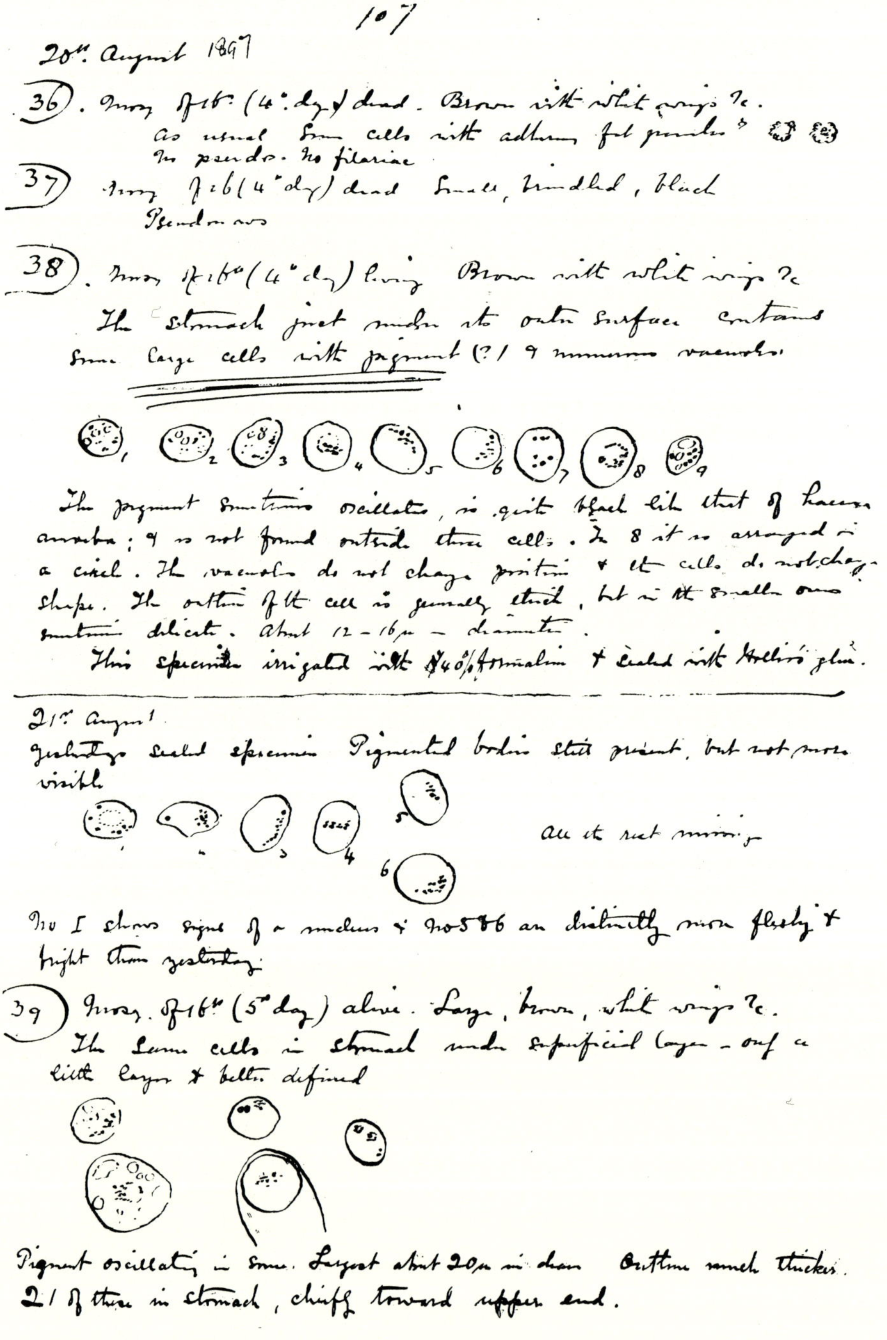

107

20th August 1897

36). Mosq. of 16th (4th day) dead. Brown with white wings &c.
As usual some cells with adherent fat granules?
No pseudo. No filariae

37) Mosq of 16 (4th day) dead. Small, brindled, black
Pseudonavs

38). Mosq of 16th (4th day) living. Brown with white wings &c
The stomach just under its outer surface contains some large cells with pigment (?) & numerous vacuoles.

1 2 3 4 5 6 7 8 9

The pigment sometimes oscillates, is quite black like that of haemamoeba; & is not found outside these cells. In 8 it is arranged in a circle. The vacuoles do not change position & the cells do not change shape. The outline of the cell is generally thick, but in the smaller ones sometimes delicate. About 12–16μ in diameter.
This specimen irrigated with 40% formalin & sealed with Hollis's glue.

21st August
Yesterday's sealed specimen. Pigmented bodies still present, but not more visible.

3 4 5 6 All the rest missing

No 1 shows signs of a nucleus & Nos 5 & 6 are distinctly more fleshy & bright than yesterday.

39) Mosq. of 16th (5th day) alive. Large, brown, white wings &c.
The same cells in stomach under superficial layer – only a little larger & better defined

Pigment oscillating in some. Largest about 20μ in diam. Outline much thicker.
21 of these in stomach, chiefly toward upper end.

Facsimile of page in laboratory notebook No 1.

PLATE V

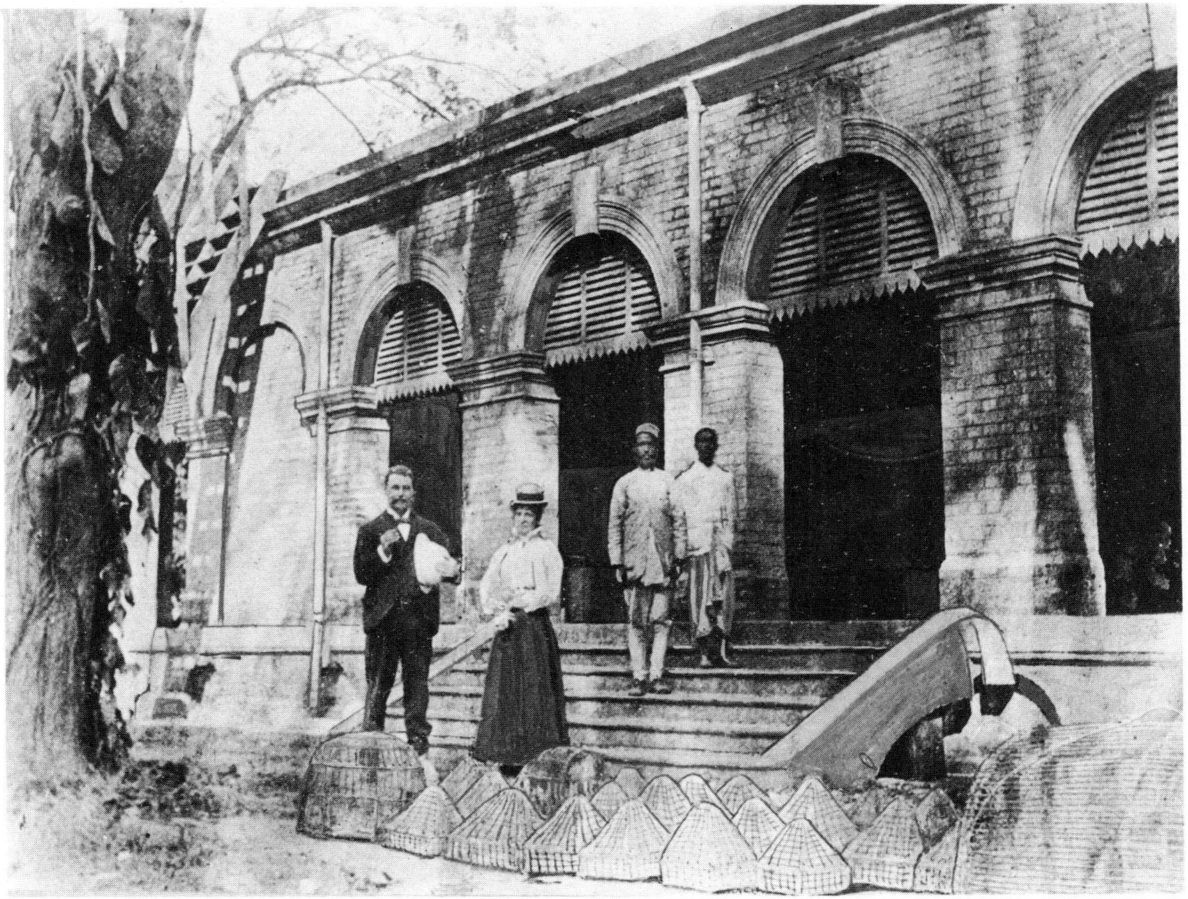

Laboratory at Calcutta. Surgeon-Major Ross, Mrs Ross, Mahomed Bux, a laboratory assistant, and birds in cages, 1898.

PLATE VI

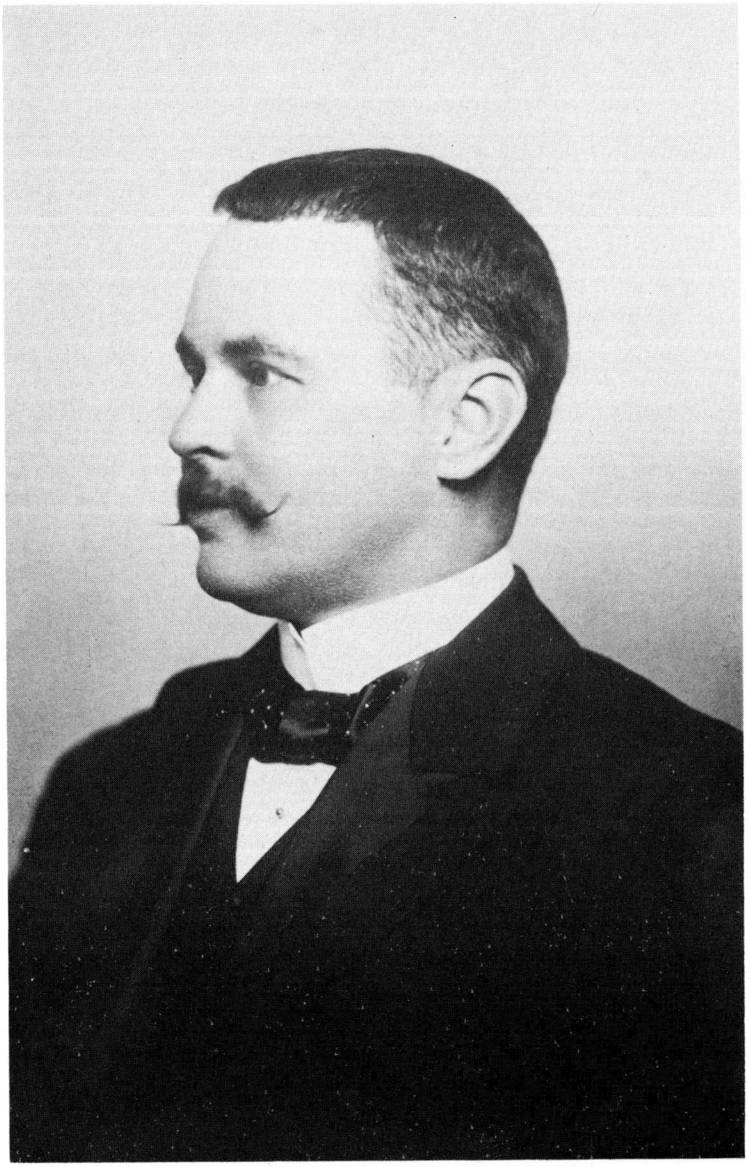

Ronald Ross, 16 November 1899.

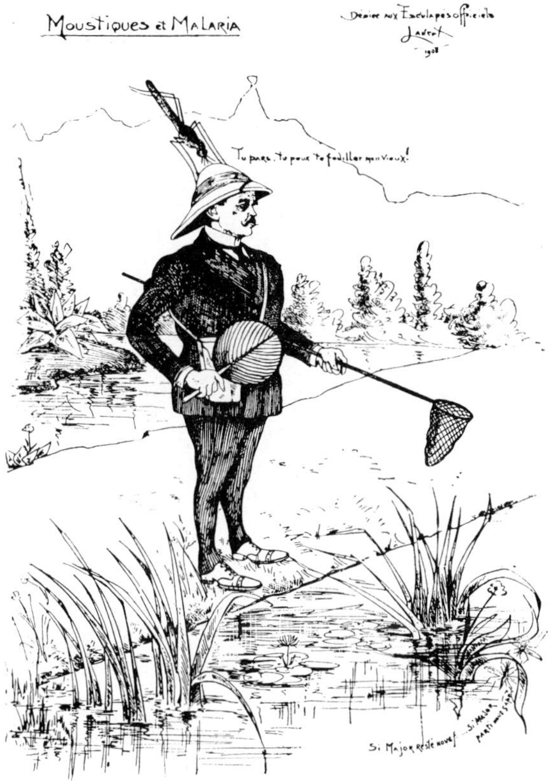

(From a Mauritian Newspaper, 1908.)

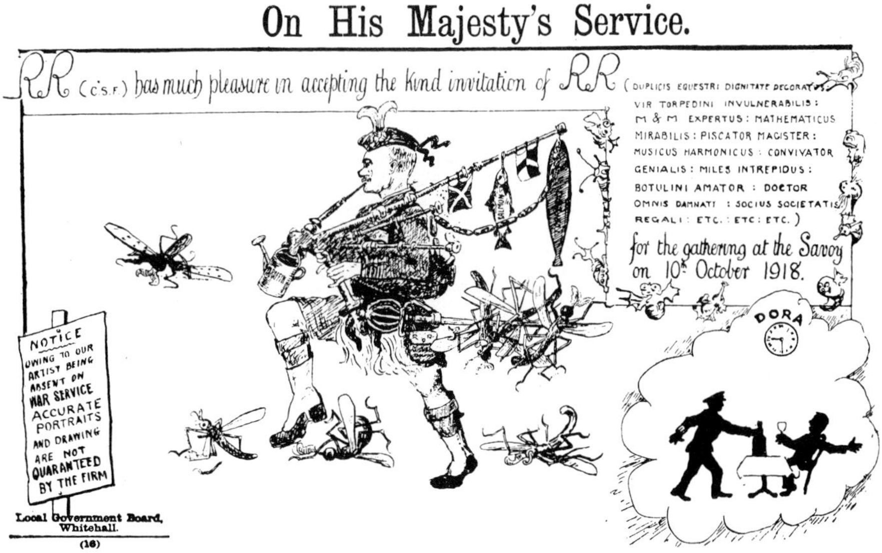

Caricature of R Ross.

great men of science made the same discovery independently of me, but I always find their claims somewhat unconvincing. I have so great a respect for this class of men that I cannot conceive them capable of the folly of ever undertaking the gamble I was guilty of! I am sure that none of them would ever have embarked on so vast and stormy a sea, would ever have been the Columbus of so wild an adventure, would ever have shown—I will not say the patience, the passion, and the poetry, but the madness required to find that uncharted treasure island! Really they have forgotten what was their true vocation—to stay at home and draw the maps after the event, to colour them red, blue, and yellow, to put their own names to the continents and islands, and to draw their salaries—a much more pleasant occupation.

But to resume—the key of the mystery had been obtained but the door still remained to be unlocked. I had found zygotes of the fourth and fifth days—but what happened afterwards? Above all, how do the mosquitoes infect men and, possibly, each other?

22 *August* 1897.

Dear Dr Manson,

In my last I told you that I was going to abandon the brindled mosquitoes for a while and attack some brown ones. Now prick up your ears because the hunt is up again. It may be a false scent, but it smells promising.

Unfortunately it turned out that my mosquitoes (brown) were very few in number, but they bit well and kept well. I dissected the first ones without any result, but some were bad dissections, broken eggs, etc. On Friday 20th I had only two left. One was very carefully dissected (fourth day after being fed on crescents). I noticed at once some cells in the stomach rather more distinct than the usual very delicate stomach cells. Altogether there were a dozen of these lying mainly towards the upper end of the organ. They varied from 12 to 16 μm in diameter and were full of stationary vacuoles. The outline was sharp but fine and not at all amoeboid, the shape spherical or ovoid, the substance rather more solid than that of the neighbouring cells. There was no contractile vesicle, but one or two of the cells seemed to be contained in some of the large gastric cells. Now I am so familiar with the mosquito's stomach that these bodies struck me at once; and you may imagine how much more struck I was when, on focusing carefully, I found that they contained *pigment indistinguishable in colour, shape, etc from that of the haemamoeba*! It was black or dark brown (not blue or yellowish or greenish like the cell granules, debris, etc), not refractive on up focusing, consisting of little balls or rods, and sometimes oscillating rapidly within a small range in parts of the cells. This pigment was not, however, copious at all and the granules did not shift their place in the cells and [?] appreciably, though I find on comparing drawings that they alter their position after 24 hours. In some cells there were pretty large clumps of pigment; in fact the latter was *exactly* and in *every detail* like the pigment of the haemamoeba.

Now what do you think of this? Well, I irrigated with formalin, sealed with glue, and labelled for you. Examining next day the cells, as I expected they would under formalin, showed more clearly and could now be made out easily with a $\frac{1}{6}$th inch [objective]. The pigment had clustered more into clumps. In fact apart from the pigment the bodies looked parasitic, though they were not nearly so bright as the coccidia I sent you from Sigur.

On the 21st I killed my last brown mosquito (5 days after being malariated) and rushed at the stomach. The very same bodies (!) only larger, more distinct, and with a thicker, perhaps double outline (sometimes). There were 21 of them, again in the oesophageal half of the stomach. The largest ones were 20 μm but some were only 12–14 μm. Pigment and vacuoles as before. Formalin etc again. I will send you the specimens when I can get some more (I want them now for comparison).

No more brown mosquitoes! In their absence, I have taken a number of brindled malariated mosquitoes [stegomyia] which I had ready and have examined them again to make sure that I had not previously overlooked the pigmented bodies. Not one in eight of them. Hence we have (provisionally): (*a*) The pigmented cells appear to exist in malariated brown mosquitoes but not in brindled ones. (*b*) They are larger on the fifth than on the fourth day. (*c*) They occupy only one part of the stomach. (*d*) They become more distinct under formalin. (*e*) They are sometimes intracellular (?). (*f*) They have pigment exactly like that of the malaria parasite.

The remarkable thing about them is undoubtedly the pigment. I have never seen this before in any mosquito (I have now examined hundreds—or a thousand). It always lies in the cells and is not scattered outside them or any other cells. In short it is as distinctive a feature of them as it is of the haemamoeba. *No other bodies but these two that I have ever seen contain such pigment; and it is the same exactly in both.* In some cells it even lies in a ring at the centre. In others marginally. In others again quite irregularly. In some cells after formalin I think I can see a central

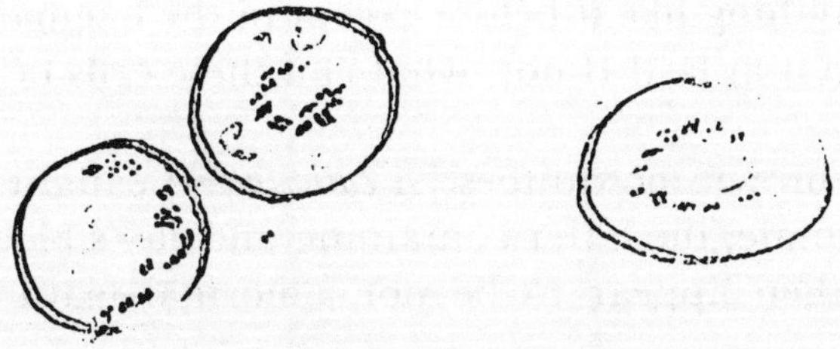

nucleus with the pigment round it. Wait now. You will say at once (as I used to think) that the parasite in the mosquito cannot have pigment because this is known to be derived from haemoglobin and the mosquito had no haemoglobin. Has it not though? Why, its stomach is full of it, and these cells which lie in the wall of the stomach, perhaps almost touching its contents, could easily absorb unlimited haemoglobin. Anyway there's the pigment, just like what we see in our old friend.

Only one difficulty remains—to get more brown mosquitoes. I may add that it is a filaria-bearing species. One of my old patients has very rare filariae and I found one kicking in the *tissues* of a 24-hour mosquito.

I must first keep my mosquitoes alive for more than five days, by giving them a second feed, in order to see whether the pigmented cells develop spores. By their appearance on the fifth day I imagine sporulation will begin at about the seventh day. If spores form the parasitic nature of the cells is established and, taken together with the pigment, leads to an obvious inference.

Next I have to see whether unfed brown mosquitoes or the same fed on healthy blood do or do not possess these cells and whether malariated ones always possess them.

All this is only a matter of a little work. Unfortunately I can't get any more of these brown devils.

Meantime the find of pigment is as encouraging as it is unexpected. It is of course quite unlikely that these cells are mere ordinary cells which have absorbed pigment granules from the stomach contents by amoeboid action. The cells are too few and the pigment too scattered and scarce—not like that of a pigmented spleen cell for instance. Besides, why should they not exist in the brindled insects?

23 Aug. No brown mosquitoes yet. Can do nothing else but look at my pigmented cells. They keep beautifully in formalin. The pigment, though much more scanty in comparison to the size of the cell, is absolutely identical in character with that of the haemamoeba. I have

never seen anything like it before except in the haemamoeba. Wonder if I am really on it at last! If not, what can these cells be? Something very unusual.

5 pm Two brown mosquitoes [*A culicifacies*] caught in hospital ward, a male and female, the latter containing one day's blood. No pigmented cells. These then appear to be not a normal feature even in brown mosquitoes.

Two points must be proved: (*a*) that the cells are parasites; (*b*) that they are malarial parasites. Please note, however, that owing to the presence of pigment (*a*) will really almost involve (*b*). Hence if I can find that the cells *sporulate* the thing is *morally* certain, though formal proof of (*b*) will be required.

24th August. No more brown mosquitoes bred from grubs but I have caught 10, one male, seven unfed females, and two females [*A culicifacies*] whose stomachs and ova show that they were fed two or three days ago. In none of these have I found pigmented cells, though all were examined most carefully. It appears then that these cells are peculiar to malariated brown mosquitoes.

With kind regards, believe me,

Yours sincerely,

R Ross.

There are several important points here. I had hitherto followed Manson in supposing that mosquitoes feed only once and then die three to five days afterwards; but I now found that I could keep them alive much longer by the simple process of feeding them again. For this purpose one had only to apply the test tube or bottle containing a mosquito to a man's skin. I also inferred rightly that the spores would be produced about the seventh day.

The "brown mosquitoes" mentioned here were of *two* kinds, both "dappled winged" anopheles. The species in which I had found the zygotes was a large, brown, brindled, and voracious species, one of which filled herself in 90 seconds off Husein Khan, but I had obtained all my examples of this species on 16 August and could obtain no others afterwards and in fact have never seen them alive again; they were probably, but not certainly, *Anopheles stephensi*.

The other species I also found for the first time on 16 August*—the

* In my Nobel Lecture it is stated that I found this small anopheles early in July or August *before* I found the large one. This error was partly due to the fact that my letter to Manson of 18 August was wrongly dated 18 July by a slip of the pen—as

single insect which was caught on the wall. But now on the 23rd and 24th they began to abound in the hospital and later even in my own house a quarter of a mile distant. They were probably *Anopheles culicifacies*, a much smaller, delicate, whitish, plain coloured insect which exasperated me by refusing to bite. They were soon swarming all over the place without annoying us and I examined numbers of them caught, fed or unfed, on the hospital walls to see if by any chance some of them contained the "pigmented cells." I find from my notebook that up to 3 September (when I went on leave) I searched at least 18 of them with negative results. At the same time I reexamined numbers of culex and stegomyia fed on malarial blood—lest I had overlooked the cells previously—but also without success. The dissection of mosquito 91 is recorded on 3 September.

SECUNDERABAD, 31 *August* 1897.

DEAR DR MANSON,

...You will be dying to know about the new cells. I have had a maddening exasperating week owing to my not finding any more of those infernal brown mosquitoes and at the end of this week I must go to Bangalore to see my wife and children. Is it not annoying?* I have had half a dozen men out hunting grubs and have obtained scores of batches—all brindled or grey. The ones I caught in the ward turn out not to be exactly the right kind, though very closely allied, being whiter and more slender [*A culicifacies*]. I cannot find where even these come from, and those caught by hand won't bite, even at night. These kinds constitute evidently a separate family of mosquitoes characterised by having dappled wings and peculiar boat-shaped eggs. I will be on them in time.

I have examined crowds of other kinds for the pigmented cells without result. I am now going methodically through a grey species with six dark grey bands on back and grey plain wings [*Culex fatigans*]. Will let you know result up to fourth day tomorrow.

Now to open my heart freely—I really believe the problem is solved, though I don't like to say so. I look at my cells daily; those of the fifth day have grown bigger than those of the fourth day; such bodies are not

I have just ascertained. I first found both species on the same date, 16 August, when they evidently began to hatch out after the heavy rain of 16 July.

* I hope my wife and children will not observe this. The interrogatory objurgation refers to the following, not to the previous, sentence.

found normally along the elementary cells of the mosquito's stomach (which are alike in all species of course); they have as yet been found only in malariated mosquitoes; above all, they contain the characteristic pigment peculiar to the malaria bug. What are we to think: what do *you* think? I fancy when you first read the word "pigment" you guessed what it was. Well now, I daren't send you these specimens for fear they spoil on the way. I will take them to Bangalore and show them all round. John Smyth is there, I think, and some other men who have got a little knowledge of the malaria bug. I'll make them write descriptions which I will send with a short note of my own to the *BMJ*.... My note to the *BMJ* will contain description of the mosquito and of the cells and will draw only such cautious references as we are as yet entitled to make. In reality—*pigment*—it is almost proof already! What else can the thing be? Mosquito's cells don't contain pigment or anything like it. I am not mistaken—it is *pigment*, absolute, unmistakable *pigment*! I have hardly restrained myself from wiring "pigment" to you but fear you would think I had gone mad. Well, I know pigment by this time. *I am on it....*

With kind regards,

Yours truly,

R Ross.

On 2 September 1897 my wife and children left Ootacamund for Bangalore, where they stayed at the West End Hotel, and I joined them there on 4 September on 10 days' station leave. My first care was to write a paper[42] on my recent discovery for publication, called "On some peculiar pigmented cells found in two mosquitoes fed on malarial blood" with note by Surgeon Major Smyth, MD, IMS. I had brought my two specimens with me and begged my friend John Smyth, a very capable civil surgeon of Madras who was then in Bangalore, to verify my finding. The article was despatched to the editor of the *British Medical Journal* between 4 and 13 September and finally appeared (undated) in the *Journal* of 18 December 1897 with Smyth's note and with excellent drawings of 11 of the pigmented cells made under Manson's direction, and with additional remarks by Manson, Dr Bland-Sutton, and Dr Thin (page 131). Here is a copy of the drawings.

It is important to note that I also described the large dapple-winged mosquitoes as best I could, saying that "the wings are light brown to white and have four dark spots on the anterior nervure.... The eggs—at least when not fully developed—are shaped curiously like ancient boats

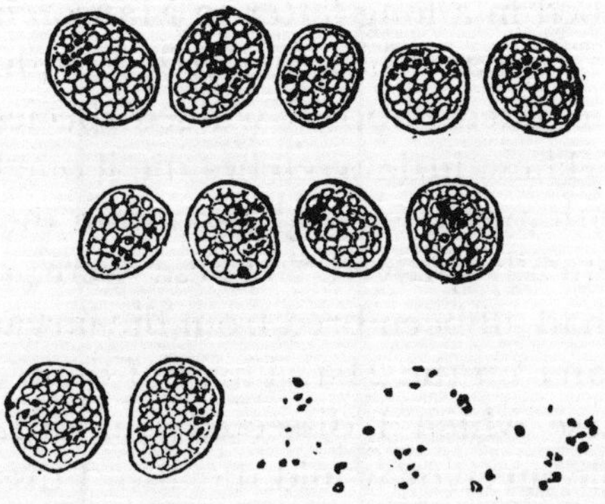

Drawings of "pigmented cells" made under Manson's direction from Ross's specimens and published in the *British Medical Journal*, 18 December 1897.

with raised stern and prow and have lines radiating from the concave border like banks of oars." Compare drawing, page 103. This description enabled the Italians to recognise the genus (Anopheles) next year (Chapter 11), as I had hoped they and others would do.

At the same time I wrote a full official report of my find to the Director General of my service and forwarded it through the proper official channel on 19 September after my return to Secunderabad on the 15th—that is, this report went directly through the Principal Medical Officer, Secunderabad, Dr Major, and the military Surgeon General at Madras, Dr McVittie. At the beginning of it I state that "the cells are in my opinion very probably the long sought alternative form of the parasite of malaria in the mosquito"—so that these gentlemen must at least have known that I *thought* I had at last found something of some trifling importance and they should perhaps have tried to help me a little.

On 13 September I sent Manson my two specimens ("worth £1000 each") with maps and full description. On return to Secunderabad on the 15th I was intensely disappointed to find that my men had secured no more of the large anopheles (*A stephensi*) and therefore started out myself to look for the larvae, hunting every pot, puddle, and pool for them. On the 21st I found hundreds of the characteristic larvae in a rainwater pool which had formed on the grass—and subsequently in similar pools and *only* in them, an important observation—but these all turned out to be the larvae of the small anopheles (*A culicifacies*). Meantime, on the 18th we had caught an old *Culex fatigans* feeding on a case of spring tertian malaria (*Plasmodium vivax*) and on the 21st it was found full of pigmented cells.

This find was described in a long letter to Manson of the same date and next day I wrote: "I have just succeeded with great difficulty in inducing four* of the allied dappled-winged species to bite a case with numerous crescents. These little wretches die if one looks at them, but if they live until the 25th and are found to contain the pigmented cells the theory will be practically proved." These were, of course, the small anopheles and they had all been bred from the larvae which I had found in the pool of rainwater on the 21st. Three of them died in the next two days and one of these which I dissected was negative. On the 24th, fearing that the single survivor would die also, I dissected it at once two days after it had been fed. It contained a number of pigmented cells, all of the same size and very small—about 8 μm, the size of a red corpuscle and of an ordinary crescent-sphere before it emits its "flagella."

I had therefore now obtained a series of four mosquitoes in which the pigmented cells increased in size according to the intervals which had elapsed after the containing insects had ingested malarial blood. The diameters of the cells were 6 μm to 8 μm at two days; 12 μm to 16 μm at four days; up to 20 μm at five days; and up to 25 μm in the *Culex fatigans*. The periods of the three first mosquitoes, as arranged here, were certain because they had all been bred from the larvae in bottles and had been fed at known times, but the period of the fourth was not certain as it only had been caught by hand, but I calculated that it may have been feeding for many days and was at least a week old (page 115).

I now had numbers of the small anopheles, all bred in bottles from the larvae, of which crowds could easily be obtained in neighbouring puddles, and I had also found that adults hatched from larvae in captivity bit more readily than those caught wild. There were many cases of malaria, both *P falciparum* and *P vivax*, in the ward and I had a number of well trained assistants and willing patients so that I calculated that in a week or two I should discover the whole life cycle of the malaria parasite, including the mode of infection. On 22 September I had written to Manson: "I shall be much disappointed if I don't get practical proof in a week's time.... A telegram to you will mean this definite announcement, and when you get it you may know that I am absolutely sure." On the same date I wrote to my wife: "I told you in my postcard that I had found those pigmented cells again and yesterday I found also some of the right kind, or very nearly the right kind, of mosquito. Today I persuaded four of them to bite a patient. I discover

* The account in my Nobel Lecture is again not quite accurate; four, not two, had fed themselves.

that this kind grows only in rainwater puddles. If these four contain the pigmented cells I think the theory will be proved. Anyway I expect to prove it completely in a fortnight or so and to telegraph home to Manson. What a fuss there will be!" On the 24th I wrote to my wife: "No more work on the germs, but I shall be disappointed if I don't finish in a fortnight. It *will* be a great thing...."

But the blow now fell; fate willed otherwise and my next letter to Manson was:

BOMBAY, 27 *September*, 1897.

DEAR DR MANSON,

I fear I must stop my malaria work at this point as I have been ordered to the front on active service. This, so far as my share in the work is concerned, is unfortunate as, when I received my orders, I hoped to complete the mosquito theory in a week or so and now I think it very unlikely that I shall be able to resume investigation for many months, if at all. Perhaps therefore I should give you a winding-up statement of my studies since I first met with the pigmented cells.

Since the 20th, when I first saw them, I have not been able to find the large brown dappled-winged mosquitoes [*A stephensi*] again. On the 18th September, however, I saw a grey mosquito [*C fatigans*] (legs and wings plain, belly nearly white, back of abdomen barred dark brown) feeding on a patient whose blood the microscope had shown to contain the mild tertian parasites. Numbers of similar mosquitoes to these, unfed or fed on blood containing crescents, had been previously examined by me and found not to contain pigmented cells. This one was secured. She was an old insect to judge by her ovaries and had, I thought, often fed on this particular patient, who slept in a corner of the ward. I kept her alive for three days more and then examined her. Her stomach contained numerous pigmented cells varying from about 10 μm to 25 μm in diameter (I have no micrometer), most of them like those formerly found in the brown mosquitoes, except that the pigment appeared to be finer, scantier, and browner, while the cells differed much in size and some of them were very large. A few of the largest cells, however, differed markedly from the others, the substance being apparently free of vacuoles and consisting of a hyaline substance in a capsule. In the centre there was a nucleus (or vacuole?) on the surface (?) of which the pigment was scattered. In the smallest cells the pigment was often oscillating just as in some forms of the haemamoeba, but in none of them did I notice any amoeboid movement.

The discovery of the cells in this mosquito immediately suggested of course that the grey mosquitoes with barred backs, though they appear immune to the summer-autumn parasite, are susceptible to the mild tertian. Proof appeared easy to obtain by feeding numbers of this species of insect on mild tertian blood and dissecting them after some days. Unfortunately I was not able to do this until the day before I left Secunderabad and the insects have all died in the train.

I was, however, a little more lucky with some of the delicate, brownish white, dappled-winged insects [*A culicifacies*] which I have already referred to as being closely allied to those in which I first found the pigmented cells. I obtained the grubs of these with great difficulty (they appear to breed only in rain puddles) and fed the imagos on crescent blood. They are wretched little creatures and die at once almost, but I managed to examine two 24 hours after feeding and one 48 hours after. In the former I could find nothing; in the latter there were a number of pigmented cells, all nearly the same size and very small, only about 8 μm in their long diameter, containing very marked and, for the size of the cell, copious pigment which sometimes oscillated and was sometimes arranged in the form of a ring. The cells themselves were so hyaline that they were scarcely visible, but there could be no doubt about the pigment, which was typical of the malaria parasite. I had no time to experiment with any more of this species.

This then closes my list of findings of pigmented cells—namely, twice in large dappled-winged mosquitoes fed on crescent blood, one in a small dappled-winged mosquito fed on crescent blood, and once in a barred-back, plain winged and legged insect fed on mild tertian blood. Of the small dappled-winged insects I have examined numbers, fed on healthy blood or unfed, without finding the cells; of the barred-back insects I have dissected as many unfed or fed on crescent blood without seeing the cells. It would appear then as if these pigmented cells are the direct result of feeding appropriate insects on appropriate kinds of malarial blood.... In the barred-back mosquito containing pigmented cells (she must have been quite a week old) the stomach contained three large clusters (40 or 50) or swarm spores, each cluster breaking up rapidly under the influence of water into a multitude of these swarm-spores of flagellulae and each flagellula almost as large as a trypanosome. All the latter then rush about in the cavity of the stomach with the ordinary movements of flagellulae. I have seen these parasites before in the malarious locality of the Sigur Ghat. The question now arises whether they are not the spores of the pigmented cells, the homologues of the ordinary flagella arising from crescents etc but which, in this case, continue the life of the parasite in external nature or perhaps are deposited on the human skin.

I must now conclude and shall do so by laying great stress on the presence of the so-called pigment in the cells. This is a substance not found in ordinary physiological cells or in ordinary protozoa, or in gregarines and coccidia, or even in the gregariniform blood parasites of reptiles; it is seen only in the haemamoeba of men and birds. What is to be said then when we now observe it in mosquitoes actually fed on blood containing haemamoebae?

Yours sincerely,
R Ross.

Probably the *Culex fatigans* had not been infected from the man with tertian malaria at all but, some days previously, from a bird containing the bird's malaria parasite, then called *Proteosoma relicta*, which proved next year to be carried by this species of mosquito. As stated above, the same insect also contained numbers of the flagellate parasites I had found in Sigur, later called Crithidia Léger, and a man to whom I gave them had fever afterwards (page 91) I therefore conjectured, reasonably enough, that these might be the spores of the zygotes—I was wrong here. The name haemamoeba was then often employed instead of plasmodium.

What had happened was this. As stated above, in June 1897 the Director General had offered me an appointment either in the Central Provinces or under the Indian Foreign Office and had later told me that he was going to give me more favourable opportunities for my investigations (page 96). If any one of these promises had been fulfilled (as I had daily been expecting them to be) I would probably have been given plenty of time to wind up my self-imposed task at Secunderabad in a proper manner and to collect my mosquitoes for identification before going elsewhere. But there was another possible development. The tribes on the Indian frontier had been giving much trouble and the Tirah campaign against the Afridis had begun so that, as I had warned Manson, I might be ordered away on active service at any time and at a moment's notice—a thing that would ruin my work just at the point of success. It was not my turn to go but that of my racing friend (page 83), who was now training horses at Secunderabad, so that I was not very apprehensive that such a calamity would befall me. But on 24 September, just after I had found the pigmented cells in the last mosquito and was gloating over this proof of the theory, the cruel Angel of Fate, who had been so kind to me before, now struck me down with the following order:

"Under instructions from Command Headquarters, Surgeon Major R Ross, IMS, will proceed immediately to Bombay for military duty."

This did not necessarily mean "active service" (which I might have enjoyed for itself) but was equally disastrous to my work. I examined some more mosquitoes and then, leaving my family at Bangalore, departed on 26 September from Secunderabad—I suppose for ever.

No sooner had I found the treasure island than I was driven away from it by an unopposable gale. I saw the promised land but was not allowed to enter it. Owing to no fault of mine two long years were to elapse before I was to see again—in another continent—that wonderful revelation of human malaria in mosquitoes. During that time all my work was to be pirated by foreigners and the same maladministration which now drove me into the wilderness was to force me finally out of India just when my discovery might have been of real help to her swarming and dying millions.

7

Punishment. Kherwara, 1897–1898

By whom and for what purpose that order was originally issued we have never been able to ascertain. Although I had just reported my new and astonishing results to my official superiors, the order was not accompanied by any intimation, official or private, as to where I was likely to be sent, what I was to do, and how long I should probably be kept away from my work. It was not even stated whether I was likely to be dispatched on active service—in which case only 80 pounds of baggage were allowed, not enough for my microscopes. The order came from the military Surgeon General at Madras (Dr McVittie) and I therefore wired privately to his secretary, whom I knew, asking for details. The answer was: "Do not know, possibly to accompany field hospital." I wired also to the Principal Medical Officer, Bombay, who replied: "Nothing known here about you." I was so stunned by the misfortune that I remember little of what occurred at the time, but believe that my Principal Medical Officer, Surgeon Colonel Major, was away and that I went to the acting commandant of my regiment and begged him to try to get me delayed for a week or two—he was a young man, much interested in my work (many more laymen than doctors were interested in it)—but could do nothing. I seem to have heard somewhere that the order had come originally from Simla and that I was to be employed at Bombay on important scientific or sanitary work and therefore wrote much more cheery letters of departure to my wife than I would otherwise have done. But I was next medically examined as to physical fitness for active service so that I left Secunderabad early in the morning of 26 September 1897 quite befogged as to my future and with the smallest possible "kit"—but with my microscope and my faithful Lutchman.

On arrival next day at Bombay I called at once on the local PMO, who was really sympathetic about my malaria work but did not know why I had been sent to him. He expected it was for active service but telegraphed to his headquarters for instructions. Next morning this good man—whose name I regret I do not remember—actually came into my room at the hotel at 7 am and told me with pleasure that I should be able to continue my malaria work because (as I wrote to my wife) "I was to go not to the front but to Rajputana. I don't know exactly what the appointment is. It seems to be half military and half residency surgeon. I arrive there tomorrow evening. The appointment is in the much coveted Rajputana Medical Service. I believe the climate will be splendid in a few weeks. Mount Abu is quite close (the hill station).... I hope you and the children will be able to come to me in a few weeks." To Manson I wrote the same day: "I shall get my residency surgeoncy, I believe, at last.... Hope to start work again immediately on arrival." The place was Kherwara. In Rajputana! Think of it: the country in which Dobson and I built our Spanish castles; my long coveted Island of Barataria!

But when I went to the adjutant general's office for my railway warrant the man there did not know where this delectable place was but found by the map that it was in the centre of a large circle of railway lines so that a long road journey from some point on the circle was required to reach it. He did not know where this point was but guessed that it might be a place called Vadnugger, near Mehsana, a long way west of Kherwara. Off we went therefore on 28 September, but on arrival next day at Mehsana I found that no transport was available from Vadnugger and that I must go by train farther round the circle to Rohera in order to get it. There I was laughed at and told that I must go to Oodeypur (Udaipur), half round the circle via Ajmir and about 400 miles away, from which I should have to proceed to Kherwara by road. I was much cheered *en route* by a happy young fellow traveller who was going, "seriously ill," to Mount Abu and who told me that Kherwara was the "unhealthiest hole in India" and was called the "convict settlement" because only officers in disgrace were ever sent there! Of course I had to pay for all the extra journey from Mehsana out of my pocket and did not recover the money for many months, and then only after much correspondence. On arrival at Oodeypur on 1 October, however, I was carried off to the residency by very kind and delightful friends, Major and Mrs Ravenshaw. He had been assistant resident at Bangalore while I was there and was now resident at Oodeypur; and, as I said, they fed me as the ravens fed Elijah in the wilderness—and I needed it because I was ill and sleepless with disappointment, not ameliorated by constant toothache! Here I received orders not to proceed—followed by orders to proceed; and at last reached Kherwara after a tonga journey of 56 miles on 7 October. It was a very small station, not even possessing a telegraph office, isolated in the midst of miles of wild country, and the headquarters of a local regiment, the Bhil Corps. The only Europeans there were the commandant, Major R A Cole, his wife and three children, the adjutant, the medical officer, and, sometimes, a missionary. I called on Major Cole at once and asked him about the residency surgeoncy. He laughed at the idea—the only thing in support of it was that the place had been under the Indian Foreign Office up to a year previously. I then said that I could at least study the malaria. He laughed again and told me that there was none there—there had not been a case in hospital for two months! In fact I had been sent all this way, about 1100 miles, merely because the medical officer, a young man of no experience, had reported sick with a small complaint which he did not know how to treat and had asked for sick leave to England on the strength of it. There was no illness in the place and his medical duties could have been easily done temporarily by an assistant surgeon or even by a hospital assistant. Was it for this that my malaria work was interrupted?

The ostensible cause for the transfer was that the Bombay medical service had been depleted by the Tirah campaign and that the Madras medical service had to help to make up the deficiency. Now I am very strong on the point that all private consideration must be suppressed in the face of public duty. But my work on malaria was not a private consideration but a matter concerned with the lives of millions of people. There were many junior officers in Madras who were not doing, and had never done, work of any importance whatever and there was my racing friend already alluded to. Why particularly was I selected for this petty job? The Surgeon General of Madras (Dr McVittie) must have issued the order a day or two after receiving my report on the finding of the pigmented cells.* I had then been working on the subject for two and a half years; numerous papers had appeared on it and I was supported by Dr Manson and the medical press. If he had disbelieved in my work why did he not question me about it, come to see my specimens, send for me to explain myself, or get someone more competent than himself to make

* I *suspect* that when the report reached him he said, "Here is the fool writing about mosquitoes again: let us give him a change of scene." I hope there may be someone still alive who can authoritatively deny this.

inquiries? If he believed in it why did he not help me? Hitherto my work had not cost the Government of India one anna. But, nevertheless, instead of helping me he now broke up my investigations; and, what is more, he must have known that he was doing so. And the civil Surgeon General at Madras (Dr Sibthorpe) was not free from blame because he might easily have helped me in many ways all this time if he had thought fit to do so.* Lastly, the Director General at Simla (Dr Cleghorn) should have taken stronger steps to redeem his promise made to me in June; but, to do him justice, I think that he tried to remedy the mistake as soon as he heard of it a few weeks later.

What most alarmed me was the experience of Surgeon Colonel W G King. In 1890 he was able greatly to improve the smallpox vaccine used by the Madras Government but the sanitary commissioner of the time was not favourable. King was deprived of his appointment and was then sent about, at short intervals, from pillar to post in India and Burma as a punishment and was nearly ruined in health and pocket. Finally, however, the matter appeared in Parliament and press at home, with the result that the said sanitary commissioner was "allowed to resign" and King was given the appointment in his place (*British Medical Journal*, 1892, 1894; *Lancet*, 1893). Naturally I thought that I was now perhaps to be subjected to a similar course of correction.

It has often been suggested that I was the victim of someone's personal animosity or of jealousy—as Surgeon Colonel W G King had been or as Mr Haffkine was to be some years later; but I scarcely think so. Thus on 28 July I had written to Manson in reply to a question of his: "No; I don't think I have a single enemy in the country. Sibthorpe doesn't love me quite, I believe—or else his manner is a very bad one—and ———, who travelled lately with Leslie, tells me that the latter did not think much of my work, malarial or sanitary.... A Madras man said to me, 'We IMS men are not meant for research and so on—we are simply doctors.' There is a certain feeling against not only research but men whose names are seen in print." The silly pose of the doctor who is above science might have been partly responsible, but the fact is that the heads of the medical services did not fully perform their duties. These expensive organisations were not made to provide sinecures for sporting gentlemen or for the do-nothings and think-nots of the

* Dr R H Elliot, who was then his secretary, tells me that the opposition did not come from him but from the military side and from Simla because the medical bigwigs there were still fast rooted in the opinion that malaria was due to a marsh miasm.

profession but to cure and to prevent disease by the best means possible. For this purpose incessant research was and is required and the heads of the services should have seen to it that every new discovery or suggestion was followed up immediately. At least they might have protected voluntary workers against unnecessary interruption and have advanced them, when they obtained good results, in preference to the scores of people of the other class who so easily obtained preferment to the best posts in the country.

Of course I was quite crushed by the disappointment and to the present day cannot remember it without indignation. For four months I was imprisoned in that place. During that time I could easily have worked out the whole life cycle of the human plasmodia in *Anopheles*, have discovered the mode of infection, and have infected healthy men (beginning with myself), just as I did with birds' malaria a year later; and I could have incriminated one, and perhaps two or more, species of *Anopheles* and have shown how to reduce them—none of which things were done in India, owing to the interruption, until years afterwards. Meantime the people of India were dying at the rate of over a million a year from malaria. The man who was officially responsible for this disaster was, I suppose, Dr McVittie, the military Surgeon General at Madras.

I made several desperate efforts to escape. On 2 October I wired from Oodeypur to the PMO, Bombay District, telling him that I had been ordered not to proceed to Kherwara and adding: "Beg you will telegraph this my application to be allowed if possible to return to my regiment or sent somewhere where I can finish mosquito malaria theory now on point of completion as lately reported to Director General IMS." On the 17th I wrote a humble letter to the same effect from Kherwara but received only the following reply from that august being Surgeon Major-General Illegible, PMO, Bombay Command (the head of the Bombay military medical service):

"I don't understand what this officer means. He was sent to this command by HE the Commander-in-Chief and here he will remain until HE orders him away."

I had already written privately to Mr J P Hewett, Secretary in the Home Department at Simla, to whom I had a letter of introduction from Sir Charles Crosthwaite of the India Office (through Dr Manson), asking whether the proposed malaria investigation by the Government of India was likely to be soon commenced, and his reply in the negative reached me when I arrived at Kherwara. So that hope was gone. On

2 November therefore I applied for the post of residency surgeon at Rewa; it was refused me. I then asked for a better paid regiment than my own—namely, the Madras Sappers and Miners at Bangalore, with which I had served in 1884. Surgeon General McVittie rejected my application. Meanwhile some of the Indian princes had long been forming a new health institute in northern India for research and I applied through Surgeon Major Owen of Patiala (page 45) for a post in it; but on 2 December I was obliged to send Manson the following post-registered telegram:

"Health institute refuses apply for my services advise you make one last effort on behalf of theory and myself if not almost certainly leave India next March if possible wire result."

On 11 December, therefore, I asked for a month's leave to go to Madras to look after my family and then to Calcutta to represent the position of the malaria work to the Government of India: the leave was refused. In fact I was imprisoned at Kherwara as securely as ever Dreyfus was in the *Île du Diable*.

Apart from the interruption of the malaria work my personal affairs were not in a wholesome condition. Owing to frequent changes of station and to the necessity of keeping my family in one place and myself in another we had been obliged to spend between 3000 and 4000 rupees above my salary, and there was no prospect of advancement in the service whatever work I did. To remain in such a position was not a "business proposition" and I decided to leave the service on the first opportunity. At the same time I wished (and intended) to finish the malaria work, and it was just possible that Dr Cleghorn might put me on special duty for the purpose before my pension was due to me (23 June 1898). Or I might be sent back to Secunderabad or might even be able to continue the malaria work at Kherwara itself in the spring. Hence I did not send in my papers at once, but in my application for one months's leave I intimated that I should have to do so.

Apart from these tribulations Kherwara would have been pleasant enough to me—a pretty little station in the midst of miniature mountains and valleys which when I arrived were covered with grass and small woods and possessed a charming little stream in which Major Cole's boys and I caught numbers of small fish like dace with the fly—they contained trypanosomes. Cole himself was a capable, kindly man; Mrs Cole was a sympathetic and hospitable lady and their large rambling bungalow was known as the "Hotel Cole." They were extremely kind to me. Even in October the climate was so cool that mosquitoes, including a few anopheles derived from larvae found in a pit, would not bite so that apart from the absence of malaria cases my work was paralysed; and later it became even cold and foggy at night. At first we had some tennis and shooting, but the adjutant and doctor soon left and for two months I was obliged to mess by myself and lived the life of a hermit. Every night a monkey wandered round my solitary bungalow making a moaning sound in the mist like that attributed to an Irish banshee. Soon the grass and the woods withered away and my stream dried up and vanished utterly like a scene in fairyland, leaving only a desert behind. At first I could do no work at all but spent my time writing letters and redrafting parts of my manuscript novel *The Revels of Orsera*; but in December I began some research on the malaria of pigeons. My article on "Pigmented cells"[42] (page 112) was not published in the *British Medical Journal* till 18 December 1897 and did not reach me till 8 January 1898. The following extracts from my letters to Manson will indicate the progress of events in regard to "the theory."

On 5 October 1897 I wrote:

"I now write to urge you to exert all your influence to get the Indian Government to take up the malaria question directly the Tirah expedition breaks up (which ought to be by Xmas). Since the subject was last mooted to government the pigmented cells have been found and it seems to me that it would be insane on the part of the government of a large tropical country like this to hesitate any longer in taking up the matter, especially as the thing can be arranged at once free of cost. Of course the government will say they have no funds after recent events, but this is no impediment. You remember that the Maharaj Rana of Dholpur and other Indian princes have come forward with funds for a health institute. If the Indian Government could see its way to mooting the point to them I believe they would subscribe at once to pay me while on special malaria duty. This would practically start the institute immediately on its protozoal side, for which a complex building and laboratory are not essential."

On 12 October I wrote:

"On examining again today my third mosquito with pigmented cells found three weeks ago I observe that the formalin has made the pigment turn into clusters of black crystals which make it appear different to what it was at first and much more bulky and distinct. * * *, the doctor here, says the crystals look like haematin ones. I tell you this to warn you that the pigment of the specimens which I sent you may have undergone a similar change so don't be surprised if their pigment differs from the descriptions of Smyth and myself and from that of the malaria parasite in man. I fancy formalin has some chemical action on pigment. My fourth mosquito does not show this change.

"You will be disappointed to hear that there is *no fever* here and I cannot go on with the work at present.... I enclose Mr Hewitt's reply to my letter asking when, if ever, government would take up the malaria subject. You observe the vast amount of interest he takes in the matter and I can only assure you again that there is scarcely a man in the government or in the department that really cares one button for all the science in the world. Many men who are doing nothing might for instance have been sent on this wild-goose chase instead of me."

In his letter to me of 22 July 1897 Manson told me that he had been appointed medical adviser to the Colonial Office and, next day, that the Secretary of State for India had written to the Viceroy about my being appointed for malaria work. His textbook on *Tropical Diseases* was finished before 11 August and on 1 October he acknowledged receiving my letters announcing the discovery of the "pigmented cells," suggested that I might have applied chemical tests to the pigment, and wondered whether the pigment might not have been merely derived from the blood in the mosquito's stomach. The *British Medical Journal* had sent him my paper. Next he wrote to me:

21 Queen Anne Street, Cavendish Square,
21 *October* 1897.

My Dear Ross,

I have been so oppressed with work lately that I have not found time to answer your last two or three letters which, I need not say, interested me acutely. You seem to be on it at last. The slides arrived a fortnight ago while I was away in Scotland on my week's holiday. I examined them at once on my return and found them in good condition enough to recognise the cells you describe. But the preservative medium was evaporating and, fearing the cells might perish, I had them drawn at once by a good artist and I hope they will appear soon in the *BMJ* along with your paper. I showed them to Thin and to Bland-Sutton, who at once recognised their likeness to the malaria parasite and the importance of your find. Personally I believe you are on the road to great discovery, but first you must be sure of where you are. Two things occur to me. The pigment in the cells may be absorbed by these bodies from free pigment in the mosquito's stomach; second, the pigment may represent an entire malaria parasite which has been bodily incorporated from the blood by the stomach cell. In either case it would not represent a phase in malaria evolution of course. These possibilities you must try to get rid of if you would choke off carpers.* I asked the editor of the *BMJ* to request Thin and Bland-Sutton to make a brief statement to the effect that they had seen your slides and that they consider your descriptions were correct. A similar statement I have made myself and I suppose these corroborative statements will appear as an appendix to your paper. I told them to hurry up with the publication.... I hope you have got a plentiful supply of mosquitoes and malaria cases and that you are now thoroughly settled down and at work again. I quite expect that ere the winter is over you will have solved the business, at all events in its main features, and that it will have been conducted so far by you that a crowd of workers will be on the details. Don't worry over them. Establish the principle and leave details to others; meanwhile move on yourself to some other big subject.

Yours sincerely,

(signed) PATRICK MANSON.

KHERWARA, RAJPUTANA, 10 *November* 1897.

DEAR DR MANSON,

I was greatly relieved at getting yours of the 21 Oct with enclosures and at hearing that the specimens had arrived all right. All I hope is that the pigment in the cells has not undergone crystallisation under formalin as in one of the specimens with me. The pigment ought to be in dots, not in rods; like this not like this. I did not apply tests for pigment because

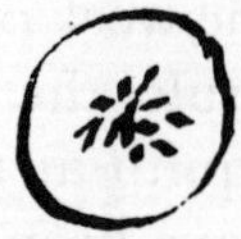

it would not do to destroy my first invaluable specimens. This and staining for nuclei etc can easily be carried out afterwards. The crystallisation of the pigment is, however, a test itself because I note that the formalin has had precisely the same action on a small residue of blood remaining in the stomach—that is, has converted it into minute black haematin crystals just like those in the cells.

Now for the view that the cells may be ordinary stomach cells which

* They were both *impossibilities*. If not, the same thing should have occurred in every "malariated" mosquito I had examined.

have absorbed and converted haemoglobin or which have incorporated entire parasites. As a matter of fact this is what I thought they might be when I first saw them, but a little reflection showed it to be extremely unlikely. If the cells be such they must be *physiological* cells—that is, *ordinary* cells of the mosquito's stomach capable of such action—and should therefore be found in all, or in a large percentage at least, of mosquitoes. Such is distinctly not the case. I have *never* seen them in hundreds of brindled malariated mosquitoes, nor in scores of barred-back mosquitoes fed on crescents or healthy blood, nor in numerous small dappled-winged mosquitoes fed on healthy blood. But I have found them in both of two large dappled-winged insects fed on crescents, in one barred-back insect fed on tertian blood, and in one of two *small* dappled-winged mosquitoes fed on crescents. This rarity of the cells precludes their being physiological and the objection is practically dealt with briefly in my paper already when I argue that the cells cannot be physiological for this reason. The thing comes under the obvious law that the constantly found cell is physiological and the exceptional cell parasitic or at least pathological. If these cells are as you suggest why are they not found in all fed mosquitoes? Besides, *do* the stomach cells take up solid particles from the stomach? On the second day of digestion the stomach is full of solid yellow particles, but I have never seen any such in the stomach cells. If the stomach cells can incorporate whole malaria parasites, why can't they incorporate whole blood corpuscles or other objects? Lastly, my pigmented cells show distinct evidences of growth in relation to the time after ingestion. They were small in the mosquito at two days, much larger in that at four days, still larger in that at five days, and largest of all and in company with large clusters of flagellulae in the mosquito at one week or so. Stomach phagocytes would not have this history. As a rule the largest physiological cells are phagocytic so that in the mosquito at the second day large instead of small pigmented cells should have been found. Then, are stomach cells ever known to be phagocytic? If so we should expect to find numbers of them filled with debris of all kinds. No, I don't think the pigmented cells are physiological but, as I said at first, the point requires formal proof. A month's work would give it. All the same the betting is, even now, thousands to one that the cells are the malaria parasite in the mosquito.

Alas for your hope that I shall have a plentiful supply of mosquitoes and cases here! None of either (or very few); the cold weather is in and the people here (Bhils) so savage and superstitious that they won't allow experiments to be made on them. I had a very slight case of tertian two days ago and some small dappled-winged insects. The fool flatly refused experiments. I don't think the insects would have bitten, though, it is too cold. People sleep here without mosquito nets.

I was quite knocked over by disappointment anent the theory when I got here and suffered from sleeplessness and neuralgia for weeks but am better after a course of fly-fishing. You must confess that it is trying to be snatched away just as one is on the point of proving a theory which one has been thinking of and working at for nearly three years, let alone being sent to a wretched place with two or three Europeans and a few itch cases and febriculae in hospital when one has every right to expect something fairly good....

Yours sincerely,
R Ross.

On 17 November I wrote:

"Another reason why the pigmented cells cannot be phagocytes is that they all contain the same number approximately of grains of pigment. If they were phagocytes some would contain a large amount of pigment, others a small amount—compare parasites with pigmented phagocytes in malarial blood.

"Many thanks for Laveran's and Simond's books, which I have received. Marchoux of Senegal has also sent me his brochure....

"By the way, it is sad to see that Laveran still sticks to that folly of the unity of the parasite. Marchoux also adopts it and Metchnikoff has gone in for it, apparently on Laveran's persuasion. What a curious argument Laveran uses. He admits that different forms of the parasite are found but says that the difference is due to climatic and similar influences. Marchoux says it is due to the resistance of some patients being greater than that of others. Not only is this quite unlikely and about as much as to say that a horse will change into a donkey if fed on thistles and kept in the proper kind of paddock but won't explain facts. I, for instance, have seen [that] at Begumpett we have tertians and remittents; close by at Hyderabad there are *quartans* and remittents. At Madras there are nearly all quartans; at Bangalore nearly all remittents with a few tertians from one locality. Fresh infections always (with the exception of rare cases of mixed parasites) show one or other of the various species. The thing is so marked out here that I personally have no doubt of plurality of species. What a lot I scribble to you! Absolutely nothing else to do...."

The paper by Simond, *L'évolution des sporozoaires du genre Coccidium*,[36] was very important. The coccidia of rabbits have "flagellate forms" very like those of malaria, and Simond suggested that the so-called flagella are really sperms (page 79). I doubted this at the moment.

On 6 and 9 December I wrote Manson long letters regarding the telegram which I had sent him on the 2nd and definitely stated that I must leave the service if not placed on special duty for a year.

On 14 December I wrote:

"I have of course been making every effort to get to work here. I fear that this is the most impossible place in India for it.... It is no go in fact. I have, however, been examining bloods of frogs, toads, fish, and numerous birds without result until today, when I got halteridium in a blue rock-pigeon (dead three hours). No flagellate forms and no fleas—but I will examine more of these birds....

"Owen's letter is a very funny one. I wish I could send it to you, but he seems to want the matter kept private. However, I think I may give you the heads of his discourse. He, Dholpur, and Haffkine seem to have had a committee meeting over my application. They won't apply for me because they think Government will put me on malaria duty. That is all well, but then Owen goes on to remark 'how fatal it is for any investigator to attract undue attention to his work at a time when the results he has to show are full of doubt and uncertainty.'* It would ruin the health institute if such an investigator should be brought on its strength and then fail. Then the solution of the malaria problem may lie in another direction to that in which I seem to believe and (he thinks) I even have an inkling of this! 'You can estimate (he says) what might be your position if such should be the case.' My ideas may possibly change when I commence real laboratory work as they did when you first showed me the malaria parasite. Then he advises me to read the 'vast literature of the subject' and above all to go and see Haffkine, if I can do so 'quietly and without attracting attention,' and he will be able to clear up many 'doubtful points.' I replied thanking him and saying that if the theory were disproved tomorrow I should have nothing to lose but that, on the contrary, the negative result would be important. I might have added that the more attention is attracted to the subject the better, even if the theory prove wrong in the end, especially in a country where every scientific problem is grossly neglected. But what

* This is an old reproach. Active investigators publish incomplete work partly to help others and partly to get back-details off their mind. Doctors who never investigate think they do it to acquire medical fame—God help us!

was the use of arguing? This is the common view in this country. If a man is enthusiastic he is advertising himself; if he takes up a subject he is a faddist and a crank; if he does not belong to some institute or other he is a mere amateur!...

"Has anyone ever been convinced by argument even to demonstration? Seldom, I believe. Men stick to their prejudices like limpets to rocks—the tighter the more one tries to pull them off.

"What alarms me about Owen's telegram and letter is the fact that he and Haffkine have great influence with the Indian Government and as they don't seem to think much of the theory and hold that it has been too much written up Government is very likely to be of the same opinion and may *very probably* abandon the malaria investigation entirely on reconsideration. I felt this strongly as soon as I got Owen's telegram and it was this which decided me to ask you to attempt one last effort. Thin's opinions about the pigmented cells will be sure to be jumped at by all of them so that I should not wonder if the discovery of those cells, so far from making Government take the matter up, will cause them to drop it *ad infinitum*."

The affair of the health institute was amusing. It was the way of the world to suppose that because Haffkine was a distinguished bacteriologist he was also an authority on malaria—which has nothing to do with bacteriology.

In his letter of 17 November Manson mentioned MacCallum's important discovery announced in "last week's *Lancet*" but did not describe it sufficiently to enable me to understand what it was about; and at Kherwara even the *Lancet* did not exist (page 142).

My next letter to Manson seems to have been that of 13 January 1898. Even then the Tirah campaign was not over and leave was still closed. I acknowledged receipt of my article[42] on the pigmented cells.* His remarks on the cells, together with those of Drs Bland-Sutton and Thin, and the notes of Dr John Smyth which I had sent (page 112) were appended to my article. Thin's remarks were very flattering to me but were otherwise worthless because he actually imagined that "the bodies in question were the ordinary epithelial cells of the mosquito's stomach containing malarial pigment"—typical example of quasiscientific

* Though its publication was much delayed I have always been very grateful to Dr Dawson Williams (Editor, *BMJ*) for taking it at all—most scientific societies and journals would have refused it. My distress at Kherwara was much enhanced by the fear that it would be rejected, that something might happen to me, and that my discovery might be entirely lost to the world.

medical opinion. I had already controverted this (it scarcely needed discussion) in my letter of 10 November and now added: "Dr Thin has fallen into a horrible pit. His needle-shaped pigment and so on in the epithelial cells are the effect of the formalin! Now I felt that this error ought to be corrected and the two other cases of pigmented cells given. So I have written a letter to the Editor *BMJ* which they may have room for." On 19 January some more remarks to the same effect are added and I said of the cells: "They are the malaria parasite in the mosquito simply because they *can't* be anything else." My second paper on the cells[43] was published on 26 February 1898 and contained an account of my third and fourth positive mosquitoes (page 115) and demolished Dr Thin's objections.

On 21 January I wrote again:

"I told you that I had found halteridium in a wild pigeon. Well, I shot several more of these birds, together with doves, finches, etc, and found halteridium in some of the first only. But none of the birds had any kind of ectoparasite—ticks, fleas, etc—though I searched them very carefully with a lens. Then I bethought me of Major Cole's tame pigeons. These are persecuted by a horrible kind of black horse fly which live among their feathers, flying out when disturbed but always returning even when the pigeon is held in the hand. They suck large quantities of blood from the poor birds, but *wild* pigeons do not have them so that it appeared scarcely likely *a priori* that the tabanus (horse flies) could be the carriers of the halteridium. But I set to work and examined 30 of the flies. The blood in the stomach when fresh contained numbers of halteridium, showing that the tame pigeons are also infected, but there were no pigmented cells in the stomach or other tissues of the flies. The histology of tabanus is just like that of culex, so that here is another argument against Thin's theory. I have also examined numbers of other Diptera—fleas, dung flies, horse flies, and a few mosquitoes—but no pigmented cells.

"The upshot of all this is that the cells cannot be any kind of physiological cell....

"PS. Jan. 26th. There are times when I think I may have been sent here as a warning not to preach 'Laveranity' so eagerly. It sounds absurd but is quite possible. When the District Principal Medical Officer came here the other day he evidently thought something was going on behind the scenes and said it was very odd that I should have been sent here. If this is the case you will probably receive an unsatisfactory answer from Surgeon General Cleghorn; and if you do I would advise the strongest possible action. Fact is I believe my health won't stand many more months of this kind of thing unless I can manage to get to work here.

"However, I hope I may be able to do so. A mosquito bit me yesterday and it is becoming much warmer. I am paying *touts* to get me malaria cases if possible in the neighbouring villages.... I am practising straining mosquito's stomachs. Am also searching for coccidia. Trypanosomes exist in the fish here, but I cannot find haemogregarines anywhere. If I cannot get to work with quartan I will try mosquitoes on halteridium."

When applying for the post at Rewa I had hinted to Leslie, Dr Cleghorn's secretary, that I should probably be forced to retire next year; and now, in his letter of 27 December, Dr Manson informed me that both he and Sir Joseph Fayrer were writing to Dr Cleghorn personally urging him to put me on special duty at once in order to avoid that happening. Cleghorn replied very nicely that he was doing his best but that I was under the orders of the Madras military medical authorities, who refused to give up their men during the Tirah operation and the plague. I am still of opinion that the discovery of the pigmented cells, if it had been put strongly enough to Government, would have enabled him to obtain my services in spite of these difficulties; and there was nothing whatever to prevent my being sent back to Secunderabad at least. But the defect of most medical administrators is that they are not strong enough to demand measures which they know are required in the public interest. At the end of January, however, the Tirah campaign was closing and on the 29th I received the joyful news by telegram:

FROM HOSPITALS, INDIA.
TO SURGEON MAJOR R ROSS, KHERWARA.

Govt India sanctions your appointment on special duty under Director General for six months rupees one thousand per mensem your transfer may be delayed. 27th January.

On 8 February I received orders to proceed. Whatever criticisms of Surgeon General Cleghorn I had made were now obliterated and I wrote and telegraphed my warmest thanks to him. We owe some gratitude to his memory.

I announced the news to Manson on 1 February and added:

"You will be further pleased to hear that I am getting to work again here,* though only with brindled mosquitoes. It became suddenly quite warm a few days ago and mosquito grubs appeared in the pots of water which I have arranged for them for the last two months. I obtained some batches of brindled insects on 29th. I suppose the eggs lie inert during the cold weather. At the same time my touts brought in a number of sick all round. Only two of these contained haemamoebae (or coccidia)—a baby with a very few crescents and man with splendid triple quartan, one parasite to 150 corpuscles. I thought the brindled mosquitoes might carry quartan. Up to date I have examined three fed on crescents and five on the quartan. No pigmented cells. I feed on the quartan both before and after the access, for comparison. A number more fed insects awaiting study. It is too cold for them to bite well.

"I am looking everywhere for barred-back and dapple-winged fellows. They are in the station for I find one occasionally in my warm bathroom. I fancy the brindled insects will be a complete failure as regards malaria—as with filariae. The secret appears to be this. The brindled species breed in *pots* of water round houses and the other species in wells and rain puddles. I shall exhaust the question of the brindled mosquitoes on quartan in few days and hope to get on with some other species too.

"2nd Feb. Three more brindled mosquitoes, one at four days and two at three days, all fed on the quartan, examined. No pigmented cells. I shall feed a number at 9 pm tonight.

"A few grubs have been obtained from an old well. Some of them may be malaria-bearing species. I believe that as soon as I get the proper kind of insect the problem will be solved; but there is the difficulty. Everything is quite dried up. I shall strain every nerve to get *proof* together before the official inquiry commences.

"You would have been amused at my shifts to persuade the quartan case to let me feed mosquitoes on him."

KHERWARA, 8 *February* 1898.

DEAR DR MANSON,

To continue my report: I have completed the research on brindled mosquitoes fed on quartan—negative. Since 29 January I have exhaustively examined 34 brindled insects fed on the case of triple quartan either before or after the access or at 9 pm. They have been

* I give the following extracts here because the Italians afterwards pretended that it was they who had done this important negative work.

examined from two to six days after feeding. No pigmented cells at all and no signs of pigment being absorbed by the stomach cells or anything like it. I think this proves that brindled mosquitoes are useless as regards quartan and crescents—as they are as regards filariae. Moreover, each of these negative results is a nail in the coffin of Dr Thin's theory. Stomach cells don't absorb solid particles from the cavity and if they did there is no reason why they should absorb spent pigment to the exclusion of other particles.

As I suspected, my pots of water all yield brindled insects, whereas three old unused wells have yielded exclusively a scanty corp of grey or barred-back mosquitoes. These, while very like brindled mosquitoes, differ from them in the shape of the egg, which is cartridge-shaped and not oval, and in the larva, which has a much longer spiracle and other peculiarities. I have a fair stock of these grey fellows and my quartan subject is still going at the rate of one parasite to 1000 corpuscles (no quinine and little fever now owing to systemic toleration); but I *cannot* get the creatures to bite. They "simply won't" as *Punch* says of Mr Balfour. They sit stupidly on the net and won't touch the patient. I have bathed him, put him in the sun to bring his flavour out, and have kept him in the net for hours during the day and also at night. No use. Imagine my exasperation. It is too cold or too dry or something. But I have fed two insects of a closely allied species caught by the hand. One contained no pigmented cells on the fifth day, the other will be examined tomorrow perhaps.

9 pm. All's well that end's well. Have just received orders to be off to Calcutta at once and report myself to the DG thanks to your action. I expected to be kept here for another two months until the war is over. Have just come from trying to feed those grey fellows. Apparently useless, but have bred a larger variety in earthenware vessels kept by me on the roof of the hospital. Will try them tomorrow.

Now comes the great time. Will prove the theory if I can. Always remember that I consider myself only your instrument in this work. You have directed the telescope; it is my part only to look through it and find the new planet.

9th Feb. No pigmented cells in the second grey mosquito. Will write as soon as I reach Calcutta. Am trying *large* grey mosquitoes. Wish me luck.

Yours very sincerely,
R Ross.

I hope this proves me to have been a duly grateful disciple.

At that time I still thought that the "swarm spores" (that is crithidia) which I had found in the Sigur Ghat and in Secunderabad might be connected with malaria but I failed to find any here. Some of the larvae which were obtained from the old well mentioned on 2 February hatched out into anopheles just before I left. Some lectures on malaria which I gave to the native officers were amusing, and, as I told my wife, "They stand round and praise me to each other in undertones. 'Isn't he a wonderful doctor sahib,' they say; 'other doctor sahibs could not do this!' They are particularly interested in seeing leucocytes eating malaria germs." But I failed utterly to persuade my hospital assistant to look through a large telescope there was in the station at the total eclipse of the sun which occurred in January. I also went twice to see the Maharawal of Dungapur who was sick—mighty but physically poor potentate—and had one day's mahseer fishing somewhere. Then, saying farewell to my good and kind friends Major and Mrs Cole and their children, I departed from that melancholy exile with a light heart and two bottles full of mosquitoes on 13 February. I spent another day with the Ravenshaws in Oodeypur, the beautiful city of lakes and palaces, the Venice of India—where, by the way, I was bitten by an anopheles (probably *Anopheles rossi*) in the residency itself—and there took train for Calcutta at 11 am. Yet another day I spent at Agra in order to see not only the superb Taj Mahal but also Mr E H Hankin in his laboratory close to it—the discoverer of the mode of purifying wells by permanganate of potassium (page 66), a great benefaction for India—and reached Calcutta on 17 February 1898.

8

The Proof. Calcutta, 1898

On arrival I found that I was to investigate not only malaria but also kala-azar, and to do both in six months! Very flattering! But the whole human race had failed to solve the malaria problem after 24 centuries' knowledge of it and the kala-azar problem is still not quite cleared up. I myself had suggested doing the latter investigation, but that was before the pigmented cells had been seen; and now I was to find that the kala-azar work was to interfere sadly with the malaria work. Moreover, I was to attack both problems single handed; not a soul in the four continents but myself was working at the malaria-mosquito theory and reports on kala-azar had been contradictory. Quite a trifling task! But, nothing daunted, this victim of official optimism cried "Victory or Westminster Abbey" and went at it. The first necessity was of course to recover the lost clue—the pigmented cells. I will allow my letters to tell the story.

8 HARRINGTON STREET, CALCUTTA,
2 *March* 1898.

DEAR DR MANSON,

I missed last mail by accident and so have a great deal to tell you by this one. I arrived on the 17th after dining with Hankin at Agra on the 15th. On calling Surgeon General Cleghorn I was told that Cunningham's laboratory has been placed at my disposal; that I am to be on special duty for six months for certain and that if necessary I am to apply for an extension; also that I am to go and work at kala-azar later on. He asked me what my plans are. I replied that it would be best for me at first to try and get on to the pigmented cells again here and that my further movements should depend on developments. I thought that kala-azar should be left until the rains but am writing Giles about it. I think you will agree with this programme. Surgeon General Cleghorn has gone [is going] home and Surgeon General Harvey acts for him. I have *carte blanche* but wish only one thing, that I had been sent back to Secunderabad for two months before the rains begin. However, 'tis a trifle.

Cunningham's laboratory is an isolated building close to a large European hospital, a native hospital, and two jails. It has all necessary appliances. For several reasons hospital patients (in other men's hospitals) are not convenient to work with. They expect treatment and the papers might talk. Hence I am starting my touting system with a constant flow of backshish [*sic*] and have been at work for a week.

Before I left Kherwara I found proteosoma and *Filaria sanguinis* in two sparrows. The large grey mosquitoes would not bite the quartan case so I brought two bottles of grubs with me. They lived all right. Much to my surprise, however, I find that the grey mosquitoes are the commonest insects here. All except one out of 19 samples have yielded this species. Brindled mosquitoes are rare and mixed with the grey mosquitoes there are a very few *black or grey dapple-winged insects*.* Close to the laboratory there is an old drain swarming with greys and a few dapple-winged fellows. The laboratory itself contains both species in swarms in dusty corners. The greys bite well here but only at night, and I hope to feed some dapple-winged tonight. I have to isolate the latter from the former by releasing all together into a mosquito net and then catching the dapple-wings in test tubes which, stopped with cotton, are the best homes for mosquitoes. I have fed a number of greys on crescents in order to repeat my former (negative) research on them; but I trust the dapple-wings will yield pigmented cells.

There is considerable difficulty in finding cases. I have obtained only four poor crescent cases and I want rich ones. Tertian is also present (two cases found) and is suitable for greys, but one case was a European who wouldn't hear of mosquitoes and the other man ran away. I hunt in the native hospital every morning before 9 am. After 10 am I see cases my touts bring me and work till 2 or 3 pm. At 7 pm or 9 pm I go back to laboratory to feed my nocturnal insects. There is comparatively very little fever here, the cases being evidently remittents of a mild type, leading to a few crescents. They say tertian begins with the first rains.

* Probably *Anopheles fuliginosus*.

Naturally there is at first some difficulty in finding cases, but I shall have plenty shortly. I have also bought some sparrows and will examine their blood tomorrow. Will try mosquitoes on them. Crombie has been very kind. Maynard has just returned from leave and will help, I think. Other men are beginning to come to the laboratory. In some quarters there is great scepticism and ignorance not only regarding malaria but other germs.

I have boys out to get me grubs from distant parts and poke about myself after them. Am flooding some ground at the laboratory to imitate a rain puddle. Weather hot and damp.

If I am not on the pigmented cells again in a week or two my language will be dreadful. Perhaps certain meteorological conditions are required before the flagella can take hold in the mosquito's cells.

Directly I arrived here I wired for my wife and children and they arrived here a few days ago. They will have to go to Darjeeling in a few weeks as it is getting hot here already.

Surgeon General Cleghorn was very brusque with me (as they say he always is)....

There is so much to be done here that I feel like Aladdin in the cave of the lamp—I can't carry away all I can lay hands on. I should like to make a methodical study of all fever cases; also to examine "eye forms"; also study *Amoeba coli* etc, not to mention animal parasites of animals. I think, however, I must resolutely set my face against wandering from the pigmented cells at present.

Imagine my disgust on arriving here to find that there is no reference medical library. I don't know what to do for some literature I want. I am writing to H K Lewis for Councilman and Lafleur on *Amoeba coli*.

3rd March. Examined two dappled-winged insects today, between third and fourth day. One had certainly been fed on crescent blood but only a little. The other was doubtful. Neither contained pigmented cells.

Only one out of eight dapple-wings bit the patient last night. I have found a child with a few tertians today. Several men are interesting themselves in getting me cases, but getting under weigh [*sic*] is difficult here. Hope to have good ones by next mail.

With kind regards,

Yours sincerely,

R Ross.

Have had letters from Dr Thin and Thornhill of Ceylon. One of my sparrows has no proteosoma.

Lieut Colonel D D Cunningham, FRS, IMS, had for many years carried out official medical investigations for the Indian Government in Calcutta, where he was also professor of physiology, but he was now at home and about to retire. His laboratory was a small isolated building containing only two rooms, offices, and a veranda and was situated in a considerable compound full of trees and bushes [Plate V]. It was to be my headquarters. There was a native laboratory assistant and a "durwan," both old men, but I find in my diary for 6 March: "Owing to difficulties in getting any work done by the laboratory assistant and durwan I have entertained from today Mahomed Bux and Purboona as assistants at Rs 8 per mensem," paid by myself of course. I chose Mahomed Bux out of about 20 applicants because he looked the most rascally of the lot and was therefore likely to have considerable intelligence!—and right well he served me. Later on he knew every bird and every mosquito and gave Indian names to some. Two old hospital beds were placed in the veranda and were furnished with holeless mosquito-nets into which numbers of larva-bred mosquitoes were liberated at night, while the birds in their cages were introduced at the same time. In the morning numbers of mosquitoes were found to have gorged themselves upon the sleeping birds by creeping under their feathers. It was Mahomed's duty to sleep on the ground between the beds in order to keep the cats away—which he did right well. His little fault was that he intoxicated himself with ganja (Indian hemp) once a week or so. Purboona was the case of crescents on which I had fed the new dappled-winged mosquitoes, but these experiments were doubtful because Purboona disappeared after he had received his month's pay and Mahomed Bux then told me that he did not remain in the net after my back was turned! Such were some of our minor difficulties.

Surgeon Major G M Giles, IMS, had reported on kala-azar and was soon to write his *Handbook of the Gnats or Mosquitoes*[44], which proved so useful afterwards. Surgeon Colonel Crombie, IMS, and Surgeon Major Maynard, IMS, were among the first students of the plasmodia in India in 1895 or before. The former was known for his classification of Indian fevers and was now a district surgeon in Calcutta; the latter told me in 1895 that he had been "working at the mosquito" and he was now ophthalmic surgeon there, but I do not remember that they subsequently published any work on malaria. I do not remember who the "other men" who came to the laboratory were, but certainly very few if any did so between that date and nearly the end of the year.

I must now explain briefly about "birds' malaria." In 1886, six years after Laveran's discovery of the plasmodia of men [page 6], Danilewsky, in Russia, discovered very similar parasites in birds and allied ones in lizards and tortoises. But he confused several kinds of these organisms and later writers were obliged to make minute descriptions and classifications. At this time most people accepted the classification of Alphonse Labbé given in his excellent essay, "Recherches zoologiques et biologiques sur les parasites endoglobulaires du sang des vertébrés" (published in the *Archives Zoologie Experimentale et Générale*, Vol II, 1894; Paris, C Reinwald *et Cie*). He divided the avian parasites of this group into two genera which he called Halteridium and Proteosoma. Both are parasites of the red corpuscles, contain "pigment," form spores within the blood vessels, and produce "flagella" when blood containing them is drawn—just as the human malaria parasites do. Since then similar parasites have been found in monkeys, bats, dogs, and squirrels, and the textbook compilers have indulged in a riot of names for the numerous different species now known. At that time, of course, no one had ever tried to find how these little creatures obtain an entrance into their hosts and B Grassi had even refused to consider the mosquito theory because, he said, mosquitoes do not bite birds. Yet the work that I was now commencing might at any time have been more easily attempted in Italy, France, America, and even London. No one seems to have studied the avian parasites in India and it is a remarkable fact that Cunningham appears never to have observed them in Calcutta, where I found almost every pigeon full of halteridium, though he actually studied pigeons' blood there for other purposes. It is stated that he was good enough to disbelieve in the malaria parasite as he did in Koch's cholera vibrio. Scepticism often saves much trouble.

On page 131 it was mentioned that in his letter of 17 November 1897 Manson had mentioned MacCallum's discovery (page 79, Plate I, figs 21, 22) to me, but in a manner which did not enable me to understand what it was. But in his of 7 February 1898 he said: "You should go over MacCallum's observations on halteridium and see if it is correct for, if correct, it is of the very greatest importance. If the polymitus* is a fertilising factor in the halteridium cycle then the flagellated body of malaria is also a fertilising factor in the plasmodium cycle. And if this is the case and the fertilised crescent-derived sphere becomes transmuted into a travelling cell-piercing vermicule† in the stomach of the mosquito

* Another name, used by Danilewsky, for the flagellate form.

† Another name, also used by Danilewsky, for the fertilised female parasite or zygote.

we have the explanation of the pigment in your mosquito stomach cells; they are carried into the cell by the vermicule. I assume you have read MacCallum's paper in the *Lancet*. This is a way of reconciling your observations and his; the one set of facts explains the other." Now in Calcutta I was able to obtain the required *Lancet* (of which he had not mentioned the number) and saw at once that his explanation of the pigmented cells was correct—they are the zygotes, the fertilised female crescents which have wandered from the stomach contents of the mosquito into its stomach wall and have fixed themselves there (Plate I, figs 23–30). I had not been able to consider the matter until this second letter reached me but now saw the full bearing of MacCallum's observation. Of itself it would not have carried us further as regards the mosquito theory. It might have helped to indicate the form of the parasite in the mosquito but not its position in the mosquito nor the kind of mosquito concerned. Indeed it would have tended to discredit the whole hypothesis by showing that the flagella are not flagellated spores and it was therefore very fortunate that I had simultaneously found the zygotes growing to a further stage in the mosquito's tissues.

Shortly after arrival in Calcutta I had written to Surgeon Major A W Alcock, IMS, head of the Indian Museum in Calcutta (now entomologist to the London School of Tropical Medicine), to inquire whether he could help me regarding the identification of mosquitoes and the literature of the subject, but he replied as follows on 18 March:

My Dear Ross,

I am sorry to have left you so long unattended to, but I have been busy with exams.

I cannot discover that anyone has worked out the mosquitoes of this part of the world. I remember, some years ago, that Dr Ranking made some observations of them, but I don't know that he published anything.

I have been looking up our photographic apparatus but cannot find anything for photomicrography....

Yours sincerely,

A Alcock.

I was more fortunate regarding the identification of the birds used by me, which were named by Surgeon Major Waddell, IMS. The crows were *Corvus splendens*, the sparrows were *Passer indica*, and the larks (short-toed) were *Calandretta dukhunensis*. To resume the letters.

8 Harrington Street, Calcutta,
9 *March* 1898.

Dear Dr Manson,

I have had rather a disappointing week. Six barred-back mosquitoes fed on tertian and five greenish dappled-winged ones fed on crescents contained no pigmented cells after from two to five days. The former experiments are open to question because the subject, a child with tertian, was in the anaemic stage and possessed, on the afternoon before the insects were fed, only medium parasites. She was so ill and was otherwise such a bad subject that I sent her away next day. The mosquitoes were fed at night and I am not sure that the child's father did not substitute himself for her. But the five dapple-wings were certainly fed on the crescent case, though only slightly. They are of the family of those in which I first found pigmented cells, but of a greenish colour.

I am having all sorts of petty difficulties at first. Cases can scarcely be obtained, though I hunt the hospitals every morning. It is, of course, the healthy season. The laboratory assistants are useless and I am training men I have hired. Dapple-wings are very scarce and have to be picked out from among thousands of greys and then bite very badly. All fed mosquitoes die in large numbers for some unknown reason. The truth is, I think, that since writing to you the temperature has fallen in a wonderful manner, quite 10 degrees. I have two blankets at night, which is wonderful for Calcutta in March. It will, however, be warm again in a few days. Perhaps the pigmented cells require a certain temperature—or rather the flagella do—before they grow in the mosquito; this may explain why they have not been found in the 11 mosquitoes here.

The question of mosquitoes biting birds is certainly settled. Three days ago I put a cage full of sparrows within a mosquito net full of mosquitoes. Next morning a number of mosquitoes were found to be fed, and on examination the blood in them contained all nucleated* corpuscles but no halteridium or proteosoma. This has been twice successfully repeated. Tonight I have six new sparrows, some of which I hope have halteridium. I am getting also other birds.

Samples of grubs continue to yield greys, large and small. I think I have made out a sound classification of Indian mosquitoes based chiefly on the shape of the eggs—namely, brindled, with round or oval

* The blood corpuscles of birds, fish, and reptiles are nucleated, those of mammals, not.

eggs; grey or barred-back, with cartridge-shaped eggs; dapple-wings, with boat-shaped eggs. There are other notable differences of course.

Many thanks for yours of the 7th February, just received. There are many facts in favour of MacCallum's theory. Perhaps you may remember I thought that the flagella may be of the nature of spermatozoa long ago.* Certainly a large number of crescents develop into spheres which do not appear to give rise to flagella. Then you may remember the observation which I mentioned to you last September [4 August 1897] when I saw several flagella attacking one leucocyte. As you say, his theory does not affect the mosquito theory. I am thinking it out and also a method for testing it.

My failure to find pigmented cells in the mosquitoes referred to is annoying as it pushes back indefinitely our prospects of obtaining complete proof shortly. It may, however, be due to coldness of weather and I shall employ an incubator shortly if necessary. My great trouble is to get tertian cases, and I have to spend hours every day in the search for them. The greenish dapple-winged mosquitoes, moreover, bite very charily and have to be put to the patient over and over again. Many of them die every day.

It *was* unfortunate my being moved from Secunderabad last September. It may be months before I get on the pigmented cells again....

Yours sincerely,

R Ross.

Congratulations about the parent of the new filaria.

8 Harrington Street, Calcutta,
15 *March* 1898.

Dear Dr Manson,

On the pigmented cells again today (in one mosquito) and have found active vermicules in mosquitoes recently fed on a crow.

Work as follows: one tertian case found (a European), who failed in getting mosquitoes off himself. Difficulties as to dapple-wings with crescent case remaining. Three more dapple-wings, however, fed on it and did not contain pigmented cells. Tertian case almost impracticable—quinine.

* I cannot find this in my previous letters to Manson and probably made the suggestion to him before I left England—but must have been overruled. T R Lewis thought that trypanosomes might be sperms (*Quart Jour Micro Soc* 1879).

Seeing these difficulties I set hard to work on birds. Numerous sparrows and larks contained no parasites. Got a new lot, also two pigeons and a crow. Had no time to examine them so, on the 11th, put them all in their cages in a net with a swarm of greys. Next day obtained about 100 fed insects which were put by to incubate; at the same time scanty halteridium was found in crow by puncture and very numerous halteridium of all stages in pigeons. The new sparrows and larks negative. Am consequently working with crow and pigeons. The former has also filariae.

On 12th also, at noon, fed a few greys, who were hungry enough to be awake, on the crow. Blood in stomach examined within an hour. Moving vermicules found at once—about six of them—also some spent pigment. The vermicules were exactly as described by MacCallum [drawing], moving about sharp end foremost. Other mosquitoes examined up to several hours after feeding showed also a few vermicules whose movement ceased apparently two hours approximately after feeding. Experiments repeated not so successfully next day. Parasites too few for such demonstrations. Obtained about 40 fed mosquitoes off crow and pigeons on night of 12–13 March. They will be examined tomorrow.

Yesterday (14th) I examined a large number of greys fed on crescent case and birds (night of 11th to 12th). All were negative. I forgot to tell you in my last that a number of greys fed on crescent case have been negative, according with former results in Secunderabad.

Today (15th) I continued examination of mosquitoes fed on all the birds three days ago [11th–12th]. All except one were negative. That one contained two pigmented cells. Of course I don't know which of the birds it bit but fancy it was the crow. The pigmented cells were in the stomach (I glance at all the tissues formally). One was about 15 μm and the other about 9 μm, each containing about 10 granules of pigment [drawings]. They were just like those formerly obtaining except that the large one had a more definite outline than those found in the four days' mosquito fed on crescents. The body of the smaller cell was almost indistinguishable but could be made out by the arrangement of pigment. The mosquito was of course grey or barred-back, of exactly the same lot as has yielded negative results so persistently with crescents, and lastly with the tertian child, but which contained large cells and swarm spores when fed on the tertian in Secunderabad.

The mere fact that only two pigmented cells were to be found in the whole stomach goes against their being physiological.

I think I am doing something wrong with my mosquitoes because

80 % of them die between 2nd and 3rd day, though I keep them in a large jar with a saucer at the bottom, dead leaves, etc.... Dead insects don't seem to contain filariae or pigmented cells to account for their death.

16th. Examined 18 mosquitoes fed on crow and two pigeons with halteridium three days ago. None contained pigmented cells. Examined also five greys fed on crescents—negative; four white pigeons, two jays, two dead blackbirds, one fever case—all negative. One of my infected pigeons contains one infected corpuscle in six; flagellates seen in it but no vermicules. Am pretty well dead beat....

Labbé is poor as regards vermicules. He thinks that nothing exists which he has not seen. Now I find that Kruse, Danilewsky, MacCallum, and others agree as to vermicules in crows and Labbé does not appear to have examined crows. Anyway they existed in my crow a day or two ago....

Owing to paucity of cases have asked Surgeon General Harvey for permission to travel to more malarious places. He says sanction of Government of India must be obtained! Just fancy! That will take some weeks.

With kind regards,

Yours truly,

R Ross.

Calcutta, 21 *March* 1898.

Dear Dr Manson,

My one wish is that you were here to share with me the pleasure which I have experienced yesterday and today in seeing your induction being verified step by step. Such pleasure comes to but few men, I fancy, though you must have felt it in regard to filaria. I am producing pigmented cells *ad libitum* by feeding grey mosquitoes on larks infected with proteosoma. This, of course, means the solution of the malaria problem.

You remember that on the 12th I obtained a number of greys fed on a crow, two pigeons, and several larks and sparrows. Out of nine of these I found pigmented cells in one only. Then I fed mosquitoes on the crow and pigeons and lastly on the crow alone and a few on the pigeons alone. Of these, 35 in all were carefully examined—no pigmented cells. Where then did the pigmented cell fellow come from in the first series? Probably from the larks and sparrows. Hitherto I had time only to examine a few of these, in which I found nothing; but now, on the 17th, I went through them more carefully, and found proteosoma Labbé in three larks and one sparrow. What then if the pigmented-cell mosquito had come from one of these? It was easy to find out. On the night of the 17th to 18th March 10 grey or barred-back mosquitoes were fed on the three larks. Excitement now rose to a high pitch. On the morning of the 20th I judged these mosquitoes to be ready. All except one were alive. I was so excited that at 8 am I could hardly dissect the first one.

It contained pigmented cells. I now had to come home for breakfast and could scarcely sit it through. When I returned at 10 am I set to work on the rest of the mosquitoes. The second and third of them contained no pigmented cells but certain peculiar pigment *clumps*. Of the remaining six, four contained more or less numerous pigmented cells—that is, pigmented cells were present in five out of the nine* greys fed on proteosoma and the rest all contained pigment clumps. This, compared with the past negative results, could be interpreted in only one way. I felt that the theory was proved.

Since the night of the 17th to 18th I have been feeding greys on the larks and the sparrows regularly. The insects have been obtained from different sources. Three out of four of those fed on 18th to 19th and two out of two of those fed 19th to 20th have had pigmented cells. Control insects out of the same bottles fed on crescents have been *quite* negative both as to cells and pigment clumps. Pigment clumps have been found in *all* the mosquitoes fed on proteosoma, in *none* of the others. What are they? We shall see very soon.

The cells are very like those derived from malaria. I will describe them exactly later. Those obtained from mosquitoes after about 38 hours are much smaller than those derived from insects after about 60 hours. Today I found a different kind of cell in a mosquito which may have bitten the sparrow. I also found *two swarm spores* in two of the insects. Let us see what I get tomorrow!

23rd March. I have not yet arrived at sporulation but have reached a growth of 40 μm after 85 hours. I find that I exist† constantly in three out of four mosquitoes fed on proteosoma and that I increase regularly in size from about 4 μm after about 30 hours to about 40 μm after about 85 hours. I find myself in large numbers in about 50% of the mosquitoes and also in small numbers in about one in two mosquitoes fed on two crows with blood parasites. I can't get mosquitoes to bite the pigeons in large numbers.

After about 48 hours many of the cells are found to be quite hyaline—that is, free from vacuoles. After 72 hours almost all the cells

* One apparently not dissected.

† I am so excited that I turn myself metaphorically into a pigmented cell!

look like spherical, almost clear bubbles and are easily seen by low powers. The pigment appears to get less and less the older the cells are until it is entirely absent sometimes after 72 hours. In most of the cells the pigment is contained in or upon a small internal sphere.

Today I watched a curious phenomenon. A specimen after 72 hours contained numerous hyaline cells; in 20 minutes they had all become vacuolated. I was beginning to think that the hyaline cells were dead and degenerate ones or that there were two kinds, hyaline and vacuolated cells. I now find that the latter are the former *post mortem*, at least with the older cells.

Of course I have only to find sporulation to complete the life history. Then I shall wire to you. I must also feed greys on healthy larks for a formality and much miscellaneous work must follow. The difficulty as regards sporulation is to keep the insects alive. Now they all die after 80 hours with the exception of one or two, though the test tubes are changed daily; but last night I fed three over again—the rest refused to bite. I am starting staining to get at the nucleus but haven't succeeded yet. Most of the insects are being mounted in formalin, as before, in series to send to you and to Laveran. I forgot to tell you that I wrote to him and had a very nice reply a few days ago. He wants specimens of pigmented cells.

Though I am working up to 8 pm I haven't had time to elaborate the best methods of mounting etc as yet. That must follow the discovery of sporulation. I want to keep my specimens this week (to look over them again) and will dispatch by next mail. I shall also send crowds of mosquitoes in glycerin.

I am endeavouring to work *backward to* the earliest forms of the parasite in the mosquito. This presents difficulties before 30 hours owing to blood in the stomach. All the questions regarding flagella, vermicules, etc ought to unroll themselves now with ease. Before this the difficulty lay in finding the proper species of mosquito because, a priori, the flagella or vermicules may be expected to die in the stomach cavity in the wrong kind.

What an ass I have been not to follow your advice before and work with birds.* Technique *much* easier. Was put off by finding nothing in Bangalore.

* I also had suggested to Manson in 1890 that he should work with birds in London, but such ideas were really too obvious to mention. I do not know why I said the technique is easier with birds: is it? I was obviously much excited when I wrote this letter.

Illustrations, photomicrographs, will be begun shortly. Healthy birds must be infected. 24th. One mosquito lived to 102 hours and was examined just now (7 am). Cells not much if at all larger but showing tendency to burst. Pigment absent from most of them. Many appearing to protrude from the outer wall of the stomach into the coelom. I think I saw signs of commencing sporulation in one or two—little oat-shaped bodies [drawing].

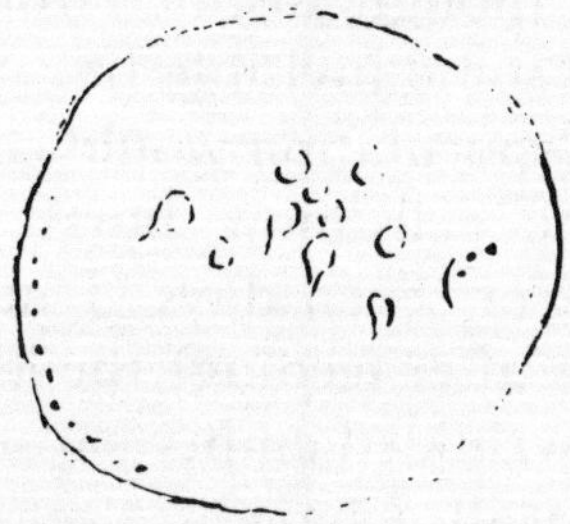

That beastly formalin has ruined many of my specimens. Hope to have time to work with other preservatives today....

Yours very sincerely,

RONALD ROSS.

UNITED SERVICE CLUB, CALCUTTA,
30 *March* 1898.

DEAR DR MANSON,

I have not wired to you only because I have not yet found sporulation, but all doubts as to the fact that we have at last succeeded in cultivating the gymnosporidia in the mosquito have vanished. I have been too fagged to write to you daily, but here is the summary of my week's work.

1. The cells continue to be found in three out of four grey mosquitoes fed on larks and sparrows with proteosoma and on crows with blood parasites (? proteosoma).

2. The cells begin to be noted certainly after one day (between 24 and 48 hours after feeding) as small bodies from 4 to 10 μm or so, profusely pigmented, lying in the stomach wall, sometimes in the external muscular coat, and apparently not intracellular. They increase steadily in size. On about the fourth day they generally lose all traces of pigment, reaching at that time a size of about 30 or 40 μm. They then begin to protrude from the external wall of the stomach into the body cavity. On the sixth day this protrusion is generally complete, the stomach having this appearance: [see Plate I, figs 25–29].

At this stage the bodies may reach nearly 60 μm when uncompressed by a cover glass; they are full of a clear fluid containing a few large vacuoles and numerous bright refractive granules, or rather globules, 1 μm in diameter and their capsule is so delicate that it easily bursts before the cover glass is imposed—which can be prevented by adding a little formalin to the water. The contents are poured out slowly *outside* the stomach. The cells, though distinct from the stomach wall, still remain attached to it by some invisible tie.

At this stage I thought sporulation would commence; on the contrary it seems to me that the cells now burst or disappear because in mosquitoes kept after six or seven days (I have examined them up to nearly 10 days, 240 hours after feeding) the largest sized cells are rarely to be found, while a few wrinkled empty capsules may often be seen still attached to the stomach wall. I have not yet determined whether these capsules are natural or are artifacts caused by the making of the specimen. It seems likely then that some trick of nature takes place at this point. The cells, either bodily or their contents only, should be found in the surrounding tissues—cellular tissues or perhaps attached to the egg. I have not found any certain sign of them yet owing to difficulties of distinguishing normal cells but have my eye on some suspicious fellows.

3. The size and appearance of the cells therefore correspond exactly with the *time after feeding* and it has been invariably found that medium and full sized cells *never* occur a short time after feeding or at any time previous to the natural time for their appearance. Hence it follows *that the growth of the cells begins at the moment of feeding and at no* time previously. Also young cells are not to be found in mosquitoes kept for three or four days without a second feed, which shows that the growth of the cells does not begin after feeding.

4. In mosquitoes which are fed a second and a third time on *infected birds, each feed is followed by a new crop of pigmented cells*—so that we may have two and even three generations proceeding in their growth side by side in the same mosquito. This proves conclusively that the origin of the cells depends upon the feed of blood.

5. No pigmented cells were found in five brindled mosquitoes fed on infected sparrows, though they existed in one out of two greys fed on the same birds at the same time.

6. I think that the cells derived from sparrow's proteosoma differ from those from crows and larks, having a thicker capsule and more scattered pigment.

7. Staining shows (*a*) that the cells take methylene blue, eosin, and logwood equally. With all, when young, I find that each cell contains a number of deeper stained bodies like bullets in a bag [see Plate I, fig 29] separate from a vacuole (?) containing or surrounded by the pigment, but as these bodies take eosin I hesitate to consider them as consisting of nucleinin. Attempts at staining only tentative as yet, of course, and the older cells are especially difficult to deal with. A capsule is well brought out by eosin and glycerin. Methylene blue causes a deep polar staining at one pole in some cases, and occasionally this masses itself into something very like a nucleus. *Certainly* the substance of a young cell contains (*a*) a capsule, (*b*) vacuoles, (*c*) pigment, (*d*) the bullet-like bodies.

8. I found no parasites in three sparrows the other day (one examination with a tired eye). Pigmented cells were found in six out of 18 greys fed on them. Hence I believe that one or more of the sparrows contain proteosoma. I have not had time to examine them again yet but will do so tomorrow.

Conclusions for the week:—

(*a*) Negative results must be obtained from healthy birds; and (*b*) there is a check where the cells leave the stomach which must be got over. There are reasons which make me think that the cells at this point give rise to a large amoeba or something of the sort which may sporulate in external nature. It is possible that this check may cause considerable delay.

I think the cells are coccidia in the mosquito, but we must wait before deciding.

I have prepared a number of specimens for you and wished to look them over before dispatching, but excitement and work fagged me so much that my eyes wouldn't hold out today and I had to go home and go to sleep all the afternoon. Feel better now, but my right eye is smarting. Anyway I will send you numbers of specimens and also mosquitoes in glycerin next week.

There is a hand-to-hand fight with Nature; she always has some nasty trick to evade me just as I am getting hold of her. But we will have it all out in a short time.

31st. The *trick* appears to be simply that I have been bursting the coccidia in making the specimen.* This morning I looked at a mosquito at the 11th day. The stomach was studded with huge coccidia, over 60 μm without cover glass. While I looked, though formalin was

* I was not using strong enough salt solution.

added, they all burst, leaving only shrivelled capsules. Unfortunately my stock of old mosquitoes is giving out.

All the above measurements have been accurately taken with ocular and stage micrometers.

I must now hurry back to work. Feel better again today after a good sleep.

Over 200 mosquitoes were fed last night. This morning [31 March] I found a fourth genus of mosquito with the most singular eggs [Panoplites, page 199]. Shall send you insects in glycerin next week.

Yours sincerely,

R Ross.

CALCUTTA, 5 *April* 1898.

DEAR DR MANSON,

I have not found sporulation only, I think, because I have not continued to look for it. On finishing my stock of 12-day-olds I thought I had been trying to rush it too much and went back a little, taking up a stock at five days. This showed me clearly that the coccidia reach full size of 60 μm and are quite extruded from the stomach on the sixth day after feeding. [Compare Plate I, fig 32 and figure on page 162]....

Well, having got so far I harked back as I wanted to occupy some important posts in my rear which I had not yet attended to. Result—formal proof of a very important question.

You remember that I had found coccidia in five out of 13 insects fed on three sparrows in whose blood I had found nothing after an imperfect examination. On the 2nd I examined the sparrows again. One contained nothing in a whole specimen; the second had a *few* proteosoma; and the third *had very many*—so many that I could not possibly have overlooked them and the bird must have been recently infected (?) This explained the coccidia and gave me a chance to make a fine experiment. I put each bird in a separate mosquito net and released on them a number of mosquitoes caught in the *same drain* and hatched out in the *same bottle.* You see the test was a perfect one as to the relation between the proteosoma and the coccidia. The insects were examined yesterday and today and I have mounted 10 from each sparrow for you, besides putting up eight whole insects from each bird in glycerin for you to make sections. (They will be sent by *next* mail.)

Results were:

Out of 15 mosquitoes fed on the healthy sparrow and examined I have not yet succeeded in finding *one single* coccidium.

Out of 19 fed on the sparrow with a few proteosoma and examined *every insect* without exception entertained coccidia and some contained fairly large numbers.

Out of 20 insects fed on the sparrow with numerous proteosoma *every one* contained coccidia and some contained swarms of them—as many as 40, 30, and so on in *one oil-immersion field*!

Thus at one stroke we get the law:

"The number of coccidia in the mosquito is proportional to the number of parasites in the blood of the birds."

The experiment is being repeated tonight. The difficulty is of course to get a perfectly healthy bird—though perfection in this respect is unnecessary so long as the law of proportion holds....

What a beautiful discovery this is! I can venture to praise it because it belongs to you, not to me. I sometimes think it is the prettiest thing in the whole range of pathology. How simple it all is after all!

I think that something funny occurs on the seventh day; hence the complete life history may not be found all at once. Of course its discovery implies the solution of the malaria problem....

I shall not wire to you until I find the complete life history. I think, however, that you can safely announce the business (if you like) when you get this letter and the specimens. Perhaps, however, better wait for my next letter though it does not require sporulation to prove that the pigmented cells are cultures of proteosoma in the mosquito.

I wish I could get a good book on coccidia—say Labbé Sur les coccidies des oiseaux (*Comptes rendus de l'Académie des Sciences*, June 1893)....

I am of course forbidden to publish on the subject until I have reported to Government, but I think some announcement should be made shortly. I will bet MacCallum will try mosquitoes in a month or two.

Yours very sincerely,
RONALD ROSS.

My letter of 12 April describes a number of specimens sent therewith, especially three series of mosquitoes fed on the three sparrows with many, few, and no proteosoma respectively. Each series consisted of the stomachs of the mosquitoes, all of which were bred in the same bottle from larvae caught in the same drain and all fed on the respective birds at the same time, and were mounted in 10% formalin. I warned Manson that the pigment in the cells might become enlarged and that my counting was imperfect because I had no movable stage and I asked him to forward the three series to Laveran, 29 Rue du Montparnasse, Paris. I also sent whole infected mosquitoes immersed in glycerin and added:

"Well, the theory is proved. Not a shadow of a doubt remains that we have found the alternative form of the gymnosporidia. The mosquito theory is a fact. The rest can be done by degrees and I want to enlarge the scope of operations. By some mistake I am not allowed to travel and they are still thinking over my request to be allowed to do so. So today I *wired* to be allowed to go to the Terai. I shall take my birds, my apparatus, and my servant Mahomed Bux, whom I have trained to the work, with me to the low hills below Darjeeling where I have ascertained there is both accommodation and fever (in the vicinity). After looking round I shall take 10 days' leave to Darjeeling, where my wife is, and get some much needed rest and exercise. The next bout will find sporulation and other things, I hope.

"I think you will agree it is time to knock off for a bit, especially as I must get fresh birds and can't hope to tackle sporulation for another week or more. I am dead beat with excitement and work. Shan't let myself work like this again at a temperature of 90 ° to 100 ° F.... I see Thin had a knock at us at the Medical Society when he talked about Roger's paper avoiding 'speculative consideration.' The Johns Hopkins Hospital *Bulletin*, December 1897, page 266, also talks about investigation guided by the 'divining rod' of preconceived idea—with very evident application to the mosquito theory.

"I think you may safely disturb the serenity of these matter-of-fact people by announcing the cultivation of proteosoma in the mosquito. Maynard will have an editorial notice of it in the May number of the *Indian Medical Gazette*. I am to report to Government on 17 May, until when I can publish nothing.... This will stop the talk about preconceived ideas. Whatever the final development of the coccidia may be, I consider the mosquito theory to be absolutely proved; and pray take this as a deliberate statement of my opinion after three years' study of the question during which, as you know, I have kept my mind open to the opposite conclusions."

Probably it would now have been an easy task to complete the life history of proteosoma at once, but three good reasons impelled me to interrupt the work for a few weeks. First I was instructed to send my chief, the Director General, an interim report giving the proof of the theory which I had obtained lest my special duty should be terminated at the end of the six months for which it was originally ordered; secondly, as there was little human malaria in Calcutta I wished to examine the conditions at the foot of the Himalayas before the rains commenced, on the lines of my work on the Sigur Ghat (and I was burning to work with the human plasmodia); thirdly, the wretched kala-azar problem worried me and there were similar diseases at the foot of the Darjeeling hills; and, lastly, I was suffering from overwork and the great heat. When my family arrived in Calcutta in February we lived at a boarding house at 8 Harrington Street, but on 24 March they had gone to Darjeeling (Ada Villa Hotel) and I stayed first at the United Service Club at Calcutta and then with Dr Maynard close to my laboratory. On 14 April, after considerable delay, Government gave me leave to travel to the Terai (the plain at the foot of hills). I therefore applied for 10 days' leave to Darjeeling in order to write my report and determined to make my headquarters afterwards at Kurseong, a little station on the mountain railway between the plains and Darjeeling from which I could descend to various parts of the Terai at will. It was hoped that I could there not only continue the work on avian malaria but also resume that on human malaria which had been so unfortunately interrupted in September 1897. Away we went therefore in a body—Lutchman, Mahomed Bux, and numbers of cages full of crows, sparrows, pigeons, and larks—to the utter amazement of the other railway passengers, European and native, who thought I was a lunatic to keep such pets.

PANKARBARI, DARJEELING DISTRICT,
3 *May* 1898.

DEAR DR MANSON,

I am rather afraid I have missed this mail but will chance it.

I left Calcutta on 17 March (April). A murrain occurred among my birds the previous night, carrying off all my proteosoma sparrows and a young crow with some kind of gymnosporidium, but I brought the rest with me. I left my man Mahomed Bux at Kurseong, 5000 feet up, with orders to find mosquitoes and have a stock up to a week or more by the end of my leave. I then went on to Darjeeling, 8000 feet (train all the way), and took my 10 days' holiday—that is, I worked only about four or five hours a day. With me I took a large stock of mosquitoes fed on proteosoma sparrows and another large stock fed on crows with halteridium. All the former had coccidia and none of the latter had. The former stock I carried to nine days. Results as before. The coccidia reached 60 on the sixth or seventh day and then no *marked* further progress (see further down). Having done this, I selected a good series for Laveran and sent them to him with a long letter and careful drawings announcing the establishment of the mosquito theory. I did not tell him about the three series A, B, and C which I sent to you as I thought you might not like to part with them, but I suggested he might write to you on the subject. I also sent you a number of greys fed on crows with halteridium and killed early next morning for sectioning for vermicules. Lastly I made a number of drawings to scale for my report as carefully as I could—the photos turned out failures. This was my holiday task. On the 28th I returned to Kurseong, where I found my man with a stock up to six days—no coccidia. He had also hunted up mosquitoes—a variety of grey (as also at Darjeeling). They bit well at Kurseong. I remained there two days trying to get sparrows—failed. Examined several little birds—negative. Examined 10 pigeons lately from the Terai (foot of the hills); *all* had halteridium badly. Some had tabanus and lice—no coccidia in these. Couldn't do much up there, so, on 1st May, I came down here.

This place is 2000 feet above sea and a few hundred above the Terai. Seems to be no fever here but plenty below. Find considerable difficulty about getting birds (which I want to carry out life history of coccidia) but hope to have some tomorrow. Shot one miner [*sic*] (bird not man)—full of some species—free forms. Mosquitoes mostly grey here just as at Kurseong and Darjeeling. Planters are getting me fever cases. There is a small hospital of four beds here. Found two ankylostomiasis cases straight off and am starting cultivating the ova according to Giles. Also a horrible case of what they call cancrum oris here. The pus was full of a huge fungus (? ray fungus), also swarms of flagellate organisms (cercomonas?), also (?) *coccidia.** Will examine tomorrow again.

I fancy discoveries are to be made here for the picking up—but must stick to my last.

Now to return to the proteosoma coccidia of the 6th–7th day. My progress is greatly hampered by want of new literature on coccidia. Leuckart and Blanchard are old and I can't get Labbé's paper on coccidia of birds. What are microsporidia among coccidia? I fancy the proteosoma coccidia are going to turn out to be of this nature and that

* I think that these bodies in ulcers had been previously mentioned by D D Cunningham and that they were possibly leishmania.

the spores will form only some days after the insect dies in the water....

Yours sincerely,
R Ross.

The letter concludes with descriptions and drawings of full-grown "coccidia"—the latter being published in two papers.[26,45]

PANKARBARI, 9 *May* 1898.

DEAR DR MANSON,

Yours of the 21st April just received. I know you are anxious for greys killed shortly after feeding on proteosoma but, will you believe it, here I have been for 10 days and can't get a single bird with that parasite. I am nearly wild. Sparrows all round and can't catch them. A few young ones and two old ones were free of it. The local idiots called Butias can't do it, I and my man have practically failed, and now I have set the police and the district magistrate on it. Fancy the whole local government trying to catch sparrows and failing! Out of 19 larks sent me from Calcutta 17 arrived dead this morning! It is simply maddening. No use shooting them of course. A planter has, however, made me a new trap and the head of the police says that if he can catch dacoits he can catch sparrows. We shall see.... You say that if only you could find a vermicule entering a cell—"Eureka," but I claim full proof already on the strength of the differential experiments plus the general structure and growth of the coccidia. I think you will admit it after seeing the specimens.

There will be no difficulty in tracing the vermicule business by ordinary dissection and washing out of the stomach,* but hitherto I have kept my mosquitoes to the second day for fear of spoiling my averages by missing the parasites so early on the first day. I have now done enough in the differential line and will go in for development on the first day and after the seventh day. Thanks for your tip about dissecting in salt water. I will use it [I had often used it already, but too weak]....

... I am making a careful study of Terai sickness, hitherto considered to be "deadly malaria." Out of half a dozen cases only one contains a few wretched small amoeboid bodies. All have swarms of ankylostome eggs besides ascaris and trichocephalus, also *Amoeba coli* and cercomonas in many. Coin me a word like *herodiasis* and you will express exactly the

* Owing to the third interruption I never had time to do this easy but interesting little piece of work.

resulting condition. It is not one parasite but many; the wretches are being literally "devoured of worms."

Now I have no doubt that a similar condition holds in kala-azar, but it is a difficult matter to say which of all these parasites is the predominating one. So far as I can see the question can only be answered after a careful preliminary examination of the chronic malaria and ankylostomiasis separately. But this will take ages.

In the meantime, if you see Surgeon General Cleghorn and he is recovered sufficiently from his accident to talk about the matter I think I would ask your discouraging my rushing off to Assam for a long time yet. The malaria problem is large enough in all conscience and is much more important than the kala-azar question. I can't do two things at once. A stock of mosquitoes is quite enough work for one day and so is a stock of patients each with half a dozen parasites, temperature to be taken (native hospital assistants are not be trusted even to do this), diet arrangements to be made, stools to be kept separate, and so on. Both will not go into one day. Let malaria be the first thing and let me do odd jobs on the rest during odd corners of time as at present. Besides, I won't be ready for kala-azar without much more careful clinical work on the Terai sickness. Remember the mass of work before me in regard to finding the species of mosquito or other suctorial second hosts for each of the gymnosporidia separately....

Have you done any more about pigment in lymphocytes?

KURSEONG, 16 *May* 1898.

DEAR DR MANSON,

I am in a vein of bad luck and haven't been able to obtain a single subject. No malaria cases. The birds which at last I was able to catch (about 20) around Punkarbari had no proteosoma and consignments of sparrows and larks from Calcutta and elsewhere arrived dead. But I have just got 15 sparrows from Calcutta and will examine tomorrow. I am consequently working all day at the report which Surgeon General Harvey told me to submit after three months. It will be called "Report on the Cultivation of Proteosoma Labbé in Grey Mosquitoes," will give full details, and be copiously illustrated with drawings to scale. I claim full proof of "Manson's mosquito theory" and solution of problem of cultivation of the gymnosporidia and hope you and Government will be satisfied with my first three months' work. On looking through my notes (which I keep very carefully, entering every observation) I find that the result of the differential experiments is absolutely conclusive.

Out of 245 grey mosquitoes fed on birds with proteosoma 178 or 72% had pigmented cells.

Out of 41 ditto fed on crescents, 154 on halteridium, 25 on a healthy sparrow, and 24 on birds with immature proteosoma, a total of 244, *not one contained a single pigmented cell.*

There is no fudge about this and only one error—that of an insect which had been left in the net after feeding on proteosoma.

The presence of pigment and the general development of the proteosoma coccidia, as I name them provisionally, complete an absolute proof. Hence I am justified in reporting (apart from orders) at this stage, especially as sporulation will properly belong to the second part of the inquiry....

Your letter of 9 April is full of business matters. You say that after the position is taken the matter should be handed over to assistants and you think you could work it through the Royal Society. Well, the position *is* taken and I think that the sooner that the affair is put on a more extended footing the better. I would suggest that, as soon as you feel satisfied of the correctness of my recent work, vigorous action be taken at once to do so. My reasons are: (*a*) my special duty lasts only until 17 August; (*b*) I may be taken ill and have to go home at any moment; (*c*) they want me to tackle kala-azar; (*d*) the work is too much for one man; (*e*) the opportunity is a grand one (and should be seized without delay) for starting some *commission* or *deputation* with some degree of permanency, to work the general subject of *animal parasitism in India.*

I urge immediate action....

Here is the programme for a Research Deputation for Indian Animal Parasitism.

Malaria carriers to be found for halteridium and each of the three species of human malaria, mosquitoes to be classified, their habits considered, their prevalence in different localities determined—an immense work. The sporulation of the coccidia, development in water if it exists, mode of infection of birds and men all to be determined and 100 other questions.

Amoeba coli, cercomonas, and perhaps *Coccidium oviforme* in men (vide Giles' report on kala-azar, which I trust)—immense subjects.

Worms, especially ascaris and ankylostoma, of intestines and filaria. To differentiate between multiple infections of many parasites is also an immense task and I believe half the sickness usually attributed to malarial cachexia is really multiple parasitism—herodism, to coin a word.

Ulcers—an unworked field almost. Parasites of animals.

Mark this, *our present system of medicine in India is antiquated, vicious, and ignorant* (as you have so often implied); it will be the duty of the deputation to reform it or attempt to do so. Our present diagnostic methods are those of the middle ages; what we call malaria, dysentery, hepatitis, malarial cachexia, and so on may be anything. Our methods of treatment are based on the treatment of the symptoms, not of the diseases. We give patients tonics, diaphoretics, quinine when we should give thymol, and astringents and dieting when the intestine remains infested with parasites. Not only our hospital assistants and our assistant surgeons but our very medical men are absolutely ignorant of the elements of tropical disease. The hospital assistant at Punkarbari had never *even heard* of ankylostomiasis, and a young medical practitioner here, who is working in a malaria and ankylostoma country, told me himself that he had never seen the malaria parasite, did not know an ankylostome egg by sight, and was quite ignorant of the worm and its effects.

If Chamberlain takes up your ideas the Government of India and the Royal Society will.

Don't ask for any *building* for a laboratory. We don't want laboratories, we want men....

Yours sincerely,
R Ross.

Kurseong, 30 *May* 1898.

Dear Dr Manson,

My work here has been brought to a full stop by the *plague scare* of which you have doubtless heard. The people, incited by wire pullers and encouraged by the extreme weakness of Government, think, or rather pretend they think, that Government wants to have them forcibly inoculated. Every medical man becomes an object of suspicion, and you can understand I am especially so. The coolies from two tea gardens near Punkarbari bolted in a body and the local magistrate and one of the planters have begged me not to work again just yet and don't like my living anywhere except at Kurseong here, at the hotel. At the same time owing to the rain it is too cold here now for mosquitoes to bite, so though

I have at last got some sparrows from Calcutta with proteosoma, I haven't been able to feed a single insect. My man Mahomed Bux is looked upon with worse suspicion than myself and in fact started the scare by shooting at sparrows near Punkarbari [page 156]. They said there is a doctor sahib shooting coolies preparatory to inoculation! I have therefore had to wire to Simla for permission to return to Calcutta but am going today to the house of a planter about 2500 feet to endeavour to feed mosquitoes....

I have carefully thought out future work and have come to the conclusion that it is *impossible* for me to attempt kala-azar yet unless I drop malaria altogether. It will only mean a similar waste of time to that which has occurred during the last six weeks. *One problem at a time*. I think then I should make every endeavour to complete the life cycle of proteosoma and work at haemamoeba as a secondary item. But kala-azar and ankylostomiasis should be dropped entirely. I think you will agree with me; *if so, will you write to that effect to Surgeon General Cleghorn*. I have already written to Surgeon General Harvey and have begged him to let me off kala-azar for the present. I don't know that he will without your backing.

As urged in my last letter I would also suggest my being put on animal parasite research on a more permanent basis as soon as possible. In my letter to Surgeon General Harvey I asked for an extension of my present duty and I hear that *Cunningham retires on the 26th June*.... Set me down specifically to solve the great problems in animal parasitism—malaria, *Amoeba coli*, ankylostomiasis, etc, etc, then I will do good work.

If I am hampered right and left I won't do good work and I think I should add that as my pension is due in three weeks I feel pretty independent. I think you will agree that backbone is necessary; my pension is my backbone and I haven't forgotten Kherwara yet. Don't want to be undisciplined at all but also don't want to be a jellyfish....

Yes, it was certainly the "pigment dung" in the coccidia which led me on to them; but I think I should have found them out without it because they are such obvious bodies on the fourth and fifth days. The whole difficulty has been not to find the mosquito phase of the parasite but to find the mosquito. In short it is a conquest not of observation but of faith. Faith carried us through all the years of negative attempts with brindled and grey mosquitoes. The fact that flagellation occurs *after* the blood is drawn was the finger that pointed always in one direction only, but the road was such a rough one that it required faith's boots to get along it. I doubt whether mere *observation* of vermicules etc would ever have done it. The vermicule found, the next thing would have been to find what became of it. Mosquitoes would have been possibly tried, and ten to one the wrong species. Result negative. The road closes here, they would have cried. But we looked up and saw the finger of *theory* still pointing the same way....

Yours sincerely,

R Ross.

My report to the Director General, entitled "Cultivation of Proteosoma Labbé in Grey Mosquitoes,"[26] was finished on and dated 21 May 1898 and was sent in from Punkarbari, Darjeeling District, on 24 May with a covering letter in which I claimed that "full proof has at last

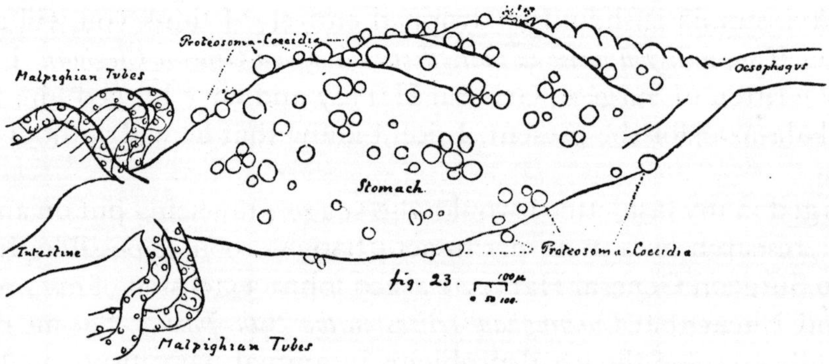

Stomach of mosquito with fully grown parasites.

been obtained, after three years' investigation, of the mosquito theory of malaria" and begged earnestly either for assistance or for release from the kala-azar duty, if only because (among other reasons) the "severe strain on the eyesight will render it a physical impossibility to continue at the same time the equally laborious malaria research." With the unconscious cruelty of stupidity or indifference both requests were rejected.* My report contained 19 foolscap pages of print, with notes of 33 different series of experiments made since 1895 and results, descriptions, discussions, technique, and nine large plates drawn by myself. The receipt of it was acknowledged by Surgeon Major Leslie and it was to be printed at once but not published without the consent of the Secretary of State in London! I subjoin one of the figures.

* Surgeon General Harvey afterwards apologised to me for this.

I communicated all the facts also to Laveran in my third letter to him dated 25 April and sent him a number of specimens.

While my report was being printed Manson, at my request, published an abstract of the work in a paper called "Surgeon Major Ronald Ross's recent investigations on the mosquito malaria theory," 18 June,[45] in which he gave the salient facts with three blocks of drawings.* He described the development of the "proteosoma coccidia," said that he wished "to place on record Ross's claims to priority in discovery," and added Laveran's statement, made to him in a letter, that "the discovery of Dr Ross appears to me, as to you, to be of very great importance.... I have shown the preparations to M Metchnikoff, who shares my opinion."

By a most singular coincidence the wide publication of these strong opinions by three of the most distinguished authorities in France and England seems to have exactly coincided with the moment when that ingenious "zoologo" Professor B Grassi, of Rome, first sallied forth into the wilderness with the fixed determination to prove the whole mosquito theory of malaria *indipendentemente da Ross*. How well he succeeded in this is one of the curiosities of the quasiscientific literature of academies and textbooks and the matter will be dealt with in Chapter 11.

For myself I hold it to be a point of personal honour to acknowledge in the warmest terms possible the help of other workers and I therefore closed my letter to Laveran of 25 April with the words:

"Will you permit me to conclude with an expression of satisfaction that after three years' labour I am at last able to make this announcement to you, who not only originated our correct knowledge of these subjects but from the first divined that the mosquito is connected with the propagation of these parasites."

And at the end of my report on the cultivation of proteosoma[26] I wrote:

"These observations prove the mosquito theory of malaria as expounded by Dr Patrick Manson and, in conclusion, I should add that I have constantly received the benefit of his advice during the inquiry. His brilliant induction so accurately indicated the true line of research that it has been my part merely to follow its direction."

Several men of science, even in India, afterwards reproached me for this last sentence, saying that it was not true and that Manson himself

* The paper contains one error, probably due to some ambiguity in one of my hurried letters. It suggests that I had found the development of halteridium as well as that of proteosoma.

should at least have attempted to realise his own speculations; one even said to me: "Let Manson praise Ross, but not Ross Manson." The fact was that at that time he had many enemies who were attacking him virulently in the medical press for having unjustifiably claimed, they said, to be physician to a certain hospital. I had not followed the controversy but attributed the attacks merely to the monkey vice of jealousy and was very indignant. I was and am a hero worshipper and he and Laveran were my heroes. He, almost alone, had helped me in the long fight and I swore to give him all the credit I may have acquired in return. So! Let the cup of gratitude spill over rather than be stinted. It is true that his induction indicated only some suctorial insect—mosquito, flea, tick, anything, that he was wrong about the flagellated spores, and that I should never have arrived further than MacCallum's discovery if I had only "followed the flagellum," as he kept on adjuring me to do. But his induction did something more: it led me to pursue the parasites from man into the suctorial insect, not vice versa as the guesses of King[15] and Bignami[30] suggested, and it kept me from wandering away into the barred wilderness of epidemiology as I almost did in 1897 and as B Grassi did now. That is why I said that it indicated the true line of research. So it did.

From this point, as will be seen, Manson's prognostications all failed. Laughing Nature showed us a miracle more wonderful than he had ever dared to imagine.

My report was in print shortly after Manson's article appeared and I sent copies to him, Laveran, Thin, John Smyth, and many others from Calcutta before the end of June.

The "plague scare" alluded to above was really a scare not against plague but against Haffkine's excellent anticholera and antiplague vaccines. These had been in use (owing to Haffkine's ability and energy) for some years, but the usual cranks and agitators now saw their opportunity and began to persuade the ignorant populace that the government were inoculating them not against plague but with plague. Numerous riots occurred and the Indian Government, which was even then beginning to show signs of weakness, seemed unable to discriminate between liberty of speech and liberty of lying, allowed the agitators full scope for their falsehoods, paralysed sanitary efforts, and thus probably permitted thousands of people to die of preventable diseases. Of course if any doctor pricked a man's finger in order to obtain a drop of his blood for examination he was thought to be inoculating plague; and even before I left Calcutta the matter had become so serious that the military

Principal Medical Officer there advised me not to touch the patients in the native military hospitals; which, with the scarcity of cases at that season, further checked my work on human malaria. When I went to the hills I found the scare established there also, and when Mahomed Bux shot a sparrow for me in a village all the coolies, some hundreds in number, on the neighbouring estate of Longview ran away in a body (page 160), costing the planters, my friends Mr J D Gwilt and Mr G C Dudgeon, some thousands of rupees! I wonder they ever forgave us. But they were always most kind and Mr Dudgeon, who was an excellent amateur entomologist, gave the drawings and description of my "grey mosquitoes" (*Culex fatigans*) which I published in my report and which I could not get from the Indian Museum.

My pleasure at returning to those great mountains, which I now saw again for the first time after the years of my early childhood, may be imagined. My work lay mostly in the gigantic trench, somewhat like the Sigur Ghat, which leads up northward from the plains to Darjeeling, richly wooded, with a torrent at the bottom of it and broken foothills on either side. Punkarbari lay low down near the west flank of it—a rest house, planters' hospital, and planters' bungalows. The railway ran up the east side of the trench and Kurseong was perched near the top of the steep declivity looking out at the plains to the south and, from a point on the road, to the eternal snows of Kinchinjunga to the north. But at that season the heights were haunted by immense clouds and even during the 10 days I spent at Darjeeling I saw the mighty mountain but once—suddenly, after a day's rain, breaking out like the phantom of another world lit by the setting sun above the rolling and grumbling legions of mist—just as my father before me painted it.

Those days were for me days of victory—spent among the magnificent mountains which are themselves symbols of victory. They stand gazing down for ever upon the plains of common earth—

> The farmyard grey with its sheaves of garner'd grain,
> The village and all its far-off cries, and the herds
> With tinkling bells,

themselves—

> Black bastions of the cloud-conquering crags,

and victors over Time and Fate. So, I thought, we poor creatures who must toil below may sometimes by our own efforts haply reach some higher summit; and during that brief holiday I planned and commenced the humble verses of mine which I love best, with a new rhythm and a rich harmony of words, my songs of triumph, *The Indian Shepherds*[40] —really the postscript to *In Exile* but never finished.

The Muse of Exile is adjured to rise from her sorrowful meditations, to ascend the mountains and to hear the songs of the shepherds there.

> Hear, mournful Muse; mute Mistress of Exile, hear;
> Sad Spirit of Solitude and of these barren briars,
> Who dwellest with tigers and serpents in this waste
> And waterless wilderness....Wake! Arise!
> Disconsolate daughter of a perisht past....
> ... Why dreamest thou thus weary
> Of drawing for ever at the deep wells of thought
> Unnourishing wisdom; weary of man and of all
> His worthless works; and not of thyself the less:
> And weary of wisdom and her lies; of love
> Her hate; of law her crime; of virtue her vice;
> And of justice her injustice: knowing not good
> If it be good, or evil if evil; o'erwrought,
> The painful reason ravelling her own clue?...
> Make haste and arise. Ascend to those uttermost peaks,
> And hear the glad songs of the Shepherds there and rejoice.

And the poem proceeds with:

> The Song of Shepherds on those Himalayan heights,
> Enormous peaks of enormous mountains that face,
> Far over all India and her silvery streams,
> Sirius and Canopus, the South and the sounding sea,
> In range over range.

9

The Mode of Infection. Calcutta, 1898

When I returned to Calcutta I knew that it was for the last stage of the great battle—the decisive victory. In April the proteosoma coccidia (zygotes) had been traced up to their growth after seven days. This seemed to be their maximum growth, for afterwards they would burst at a touch on the cover glass. They were evidently ripe, yet when they burst nothing very visible came forth. I dissected mosquitoes in plain tap water or in "normal saline" (a weak, 0·4% solution of salt) and preferred the former because it made the *young* zygotes more visible. Manson had recently suggested the latter, thinking that I had not been employing it, and this suggestion gave me another idea: that a *much stronger* salt solution should reveal the contents of the *ripe* zygotes.

CALCUTTA (CARE OF POSTMASTER, CALCUTTA),
13 *June* 1898.

DEAR DR MANSON,

As anticipated in my last I was obliged to return to this place owing to difficulties in getting birds with proteosoma and in persuading mosquitoes to bite at Kurseong and Punkarbari. I arrived here on the 4th. Owing to plague scare all the bird catchers had bolted and my sparrows from Kurseong died on returning (to their own climate!) so that I had some difficulties in getting under weigh [*sic*], again. At last, however, I have some beautiful stock of proteosoma-bearing greys and shall be hard at sporulation in three more days. The plan I shall adopt will be to examine only dead insects as, all considered, I think the spores will form some time after death. At the same time I have a number of healthy young birds which I will try to infect by cramming malariated mosquitoes down their throats.* I have just ascertained beyond a doubt that birds eat mosquitoes. Out of 70 which I tried to refeed last night only about 50 were found in the net (a new one) this morning.

The difficulties are minor ones—the birds are killed by too many mosquitoes, the insects die in numbers at each refeed and when they lay their eggs. There is also difficulty in getting numerous sparrows here at present. But it is quite possible I may complete the life cycle of proteosoma in a few weeks.

I am also getting dapple-wings [*Anopheles rossi*] in large numbers now in *rainwater puddles*. These I am going to try on halteridium. Of course I am not allowed to experiment on human beings here because of the scare—at least just yet....

Surgeon General Harvey has ordered 100 copies of my report, which is being run through the press as soon as possible. The plates are to be photolithographed. I hope it will arrive in ample time for the July meeting [of the British Medical Association]. He has, however, refused to *publish* the report, though he says I may send copies to experts....

14th June. Nearly 30 of my best stock died last night. It is a beautiful stock, every mosquito having numerous coccidia. Also my best sparrows gave up the ghost. Owing to the heat, I expect, the coccidia in the dead mosquitoes are unusually large for the period—fourth day reaching 45 μm, some of them, and protruding freely. Hence I have left 20 of the dead insects to rot in water with a view to seeing what becomes of the coccidia. Sporulation *may* take place before complete growth, as in birds' proteosoma....

I fear I have lost time in going to the Terai but hardly expected the sparrows there to have no proteosoma nor to be hindered by the plague scare. I might have finished proteosoma here and then come home for the Tropical Section. Anyway it is possible I may be home in September or so if I can infect birds.

I applied for assistance. Refused of course. Things will never be done on a proper scale until a fuss has been made....

Yours sincerely,
R Ross.

* These experiments were to verify Manson's conjectures that the plasmodia would now enter the water in which mosquitoes containing them had died or would be swallowed as "mosquito-dust."

CALCUTTA, 22 *June* 1898.

DEAR DR MANSON,

...I think I am on the verge of another great advance. I have kept dead mosquitoes until they have fallen to bits—no development of the coccidia of fourth to seventh days. They resist longer than the stomach tissues but evidently degenerate—capsule shrinks, contents contract and become yellow, and ultimately bacteria enter. In the last stage of decomposition the stomach consists of a bag, the outer coat, full of bacteria and having empty capsules of coccidia attached to it on the outside [see Manson's speculation, page 14].

Hence no opening here apparently. Next the former suspicion is being confirmed that the coccidia burst in the *living insect* on about the seventh or eighth day because in insects after that date (when fed only for the *first time* on proteosoma blood) only empty capsules seem to occur [Plate I, figs 33, 34].

But I have found a most useful reagent—fairly strong salt solution. This brings out in a wonderful manner the *striation* of a coccidia and makes them look like caterpillars contained in an egg. Is it karyokinesis?

No, I think it likely that the striations are due to the coccidia, or some of them, being packed full of *germinal threads* 10 μm in length which are *scattered into the living insect's coelom.* I say this on the experience of one insect only of eighth day examined this morning. It contained many mature proteosoma coccidia deeply striated and also swarms of small bodies [drawing—see figure, page 171] *feebly moving* in the salt solution and evidently escaped from the body cavity of the insect. I thought that by pressure I could force similar bodies out of the coccidia. The bodies are not bacteria; they taper at both ends and are broader in the centre, which appears capable of some change of shape.

23rd. Have just found the "germinal rods" again in a mosquito of eighth day whose stomach was covered with empty capsules. Think I am on the track and hope to give you definite news by next mail.

I have heard from Laveran; the specimens I sent him have not arrived though I registered the parcel....

Yours sincerely,
R ROSS.

It had been arranged that a new section for tropical medicine was to be created at future annual meetings of the British Medical Association. The first of these was to be held at Edinburgh near the end of July and

Manson was to be the first president of the section. I was straining every nerve to send him specimens and to complete the life cycle before that date—as in fact I did. I wrote to Manson on 28 June 1898 as follows:

CALCUTTA, 28 *June* 1898.

DEAR DR MANSON,

I dispatched some copies of my report to you by this mail with one for Sir J Fayrer. Will you oblige me greatly by sending it on to him? I don't know his address but will write to him as well. I fear much I shan't be able to send you good second-day specimens as my infected birds are so much better that they don't yield good crops any longer but will try tomorrow.

The bulk of the copies of my report are not sewn even yet and will never reach the Secretary of State through the Government of India in time for the BMA meeting. The only thing to be done then is for you to send one of the copies I have dispatched to you with Leslie's letter and ask his permission to publish. He is sure to give it straight off.

Another advance has been made. On the sixth and seventh days the coccidia form a large number of germinal rods (?) 12 μm in length. This is easily seen by using a rather strong salt solution, which gives many of the coccidia from fifth day a striated appearance as figures in the report but more marked. By using pressure these coccidia are easily burst, when the rods pour out.

They are just about 12 μm in length and all the same size. They taper toward each end and are therefore thicker in the middle. In salt solution after a time they show one or more vacuoles in the middle part and become bent angularly. They stain easily with Loeffler, Delafield, etc and then show one or more chromatin granules toward the middle, between the vacuoles, and the same time become broader, when they look very like small trypanosomes. They often possess swellings somewhere along their length, very like flagella do. On addition of water they tend to curl up and look like granular material. I am not sure whether they are at all motile, though I have often thought so. I think especially that they bend and straighten themselves, but these points are difficult to make out because of their continual Brownian movement, while it is evident that both water and salt solutions kill them.

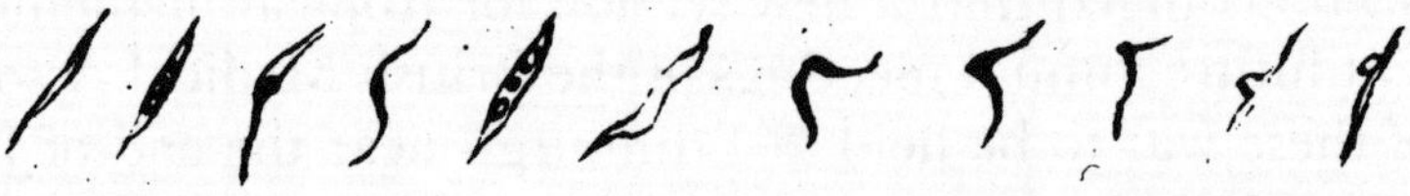

When youngish striated coccidia are burst these bodies issue attached like rays to circular cells [see Plate I, fig 31] and others similar.

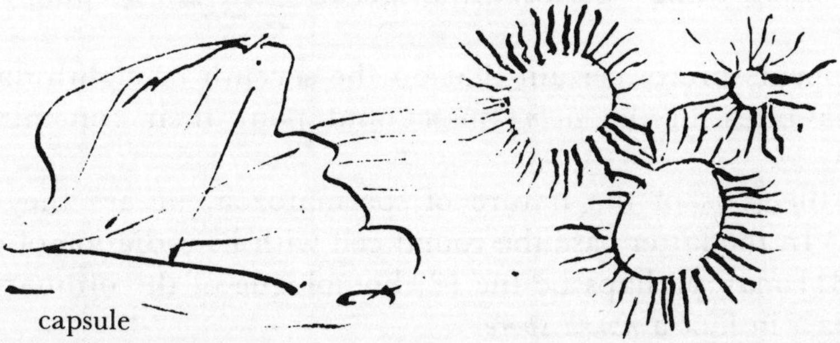

This arrangement can often be seen within the unburst coccidium. The circular cells to which the germinal rods are attached stain easily, like the rods, but show no nucleus.

In older coccidia the rods pour out all separately and the cells are not to be found.

The rods are easily seen in large numbers in eight-day mosquitoes (and earlier) all round the stomach and amongst the abdominal scales. They are in the coelom.

The use of fairly strong salt solution has enabled me to ascertain these points, which may be taken as quite certain.

No development of the rods has yet been observed either in living or in decomposing mosquitoes.

One never finds all the coccidia, even when mature, to be striated—that is, to contain rods. The rest seem to contain nothing but a clear fluid with bright oil globules.

I have searched in vain in living mosquitoes and dead ones for anything like psorosperms or pseudonavicellae unless the black sausage-

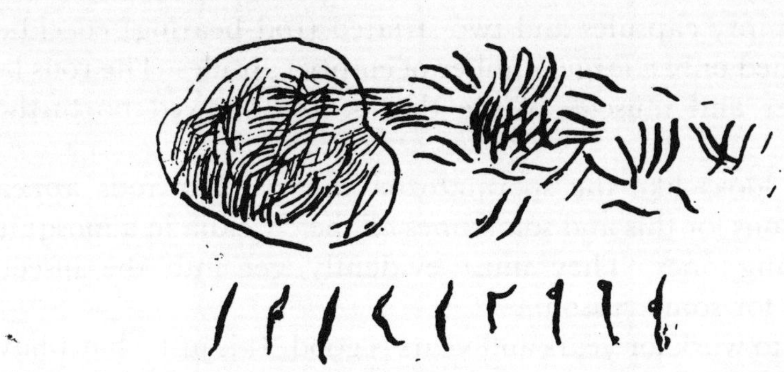

"Germinal rods" pouring out of a mature "coccidium." From letter of Ross to Laveran, 18 July 1898.

shaped bodies [Plate I, fig 34] are such. These, however, are only rarely seen and appear then to exist only in empty capsules. I expect they are fungi or something—germs within germs—but am keeping my eye on them.*

It appears pretty certain that on the seventh or eighth days all the coccidia burst in the *living* insect and pour their contents into the coelom.

Are the rods of the nature of spermatozoa, or are they falciform bodies? In the latter case the round cell with its radiation of rod [Plate I, fig 31] may perhaps be the [?] homologue of the ordinary spore of coccidia—in fact a *naked spore*.

Nature probably makes some extraordinary effort here in order to complete the life cycle. What the dickens she is going to do next I cannot imagine at all. Great difficulties may, however, be feared owing to the absence of hard spores. But I am trying to turn the position by blind attempts to infect healthy sparrows.

Infected mosquitoes have been fed on five healthy sparrows for a fortnight. On examining again the other day a few proteosoma were found in one of the sparrows—scarcely good enough. I am therefore feeding three healthy sparrows with mosquitoes containing mature coccidia. [Still trying to verify Manson's conjectures.]

But this climate! I can perhaps stand another month of it. It is hell, simply; and the constant strain on mind and eye at this temperature is making me thoroughly ill. If I cannot infect birds or find a clear opening by the end of July I *must* clear out. Permanent work here is out of the question for me, I feel. But I shall stick on to the last gasp in order to be able to wire to you before the BMA meeting if possible....

29th June. I have found large numbers of germinal rods in the thorax of two mosquitoes, one a *six*-day and one an *eight*-day one. The former contained two empty capsules and two striated (rod-bearing) coccidia; the latter contained only a large number of empty capsules. The rods lay among the scales and muscles of the thorax and showed no further development.

This scarcely looks like the spermatozoa theory. The rods appear much too numerous for this and sometimes *all* the coccidia in a mosquito are rod-containing ones. They must evidently get into the insect's circulating fluid for some reason....

Thin's advice to work for years and years is good. It is just what I have

* This is what they proved likely to be—after much questioning and research (page 202).

done. It is also good not to publish until there is not a vestige of objection possible. Here again the report follows his advice.

My advice is that any further objections are scarcely to be recommended as they will meet with a terrible fate, I think. I don't see any line of criticism which can be taken up against the theory with any chance of success. I venture to say that there is no fact in the life history of any parasite more certain than that proteosoma in the bird becomes coccidium* in the mosquito. It is quite certain. The man who criticises will die; he will knock his head against a rock.

Many thanks for your efforts on behalf of a commission. Remember always that the Government of India is a *mule* as regards science. It won't do anything unless driven. As for the IMS, it does not care a cent for the whole business. Remember also that if the Government of India won't do anything I am always willing (if not anxious) to take my pension and work elsewhere and for other masters. What do you think of Egypt?...

CALCUTTA, 6 *July* 1898.

DEAR DR MANSON,

Let me in the first place felicitate you and the profession on the new tropical section and let me wish it every success in the future. It is started under the best possible auspices.

I hope this letter will reach you at Edinborough [*sic*]. If so it will be opportune because I feel *almost* justified in saying that I have completed the life cycle, or rather perhaps one life cycle, of proteosoma and therefore in all probability of the malaria parasite. I say "almost" because though I think I have seized the final position, I have not yet occupied it with my full forces.

My last letter left me face to face with the astonishing fact that the germinal rods were to be found in the thorax as well as in the abdomen. Instead of the hard resisting spores we expected to arrive at—spores easily seen and followed—here were a multitude of delicate little threads, scarcely more visible than dead flagella and poured out amongst the million objects which, under an oil-immersion lens, go to make up a mosquito. I dare say you imagined my consternation. I could not conceive what was to happen to the rods.

Well, I was in for a battle. It was, I think, the last stand—on the very breathless heights of science. I am nearly blind and deaf with

* Of course the term coccidium here is merely provisional. I meant coccidium-like bodies. Obviously I had no time to consider mere names.

exhaustion!!—but triumphant. Expect one of the most wonderful things.

The rods were evidently in the insect's *blood*. By merely pricking the back of the thorax and letting the milky juice flow into a minute drop of salt solution thousands of proteosoma coccidium rods could easily be obtained. The question was what next?

I now divided my insects before dissection between the thorax and abdomen and examined each part separately. It was found that the rods were often *more numerous in the thorax than in the abdomen*; there were even cases where scarcely one could be found in the abdomen (the coccidia having evidently burst some days previously as shown by their empty capsules), while numbers (four or five in a field) could be detected on tearing up the thorax and head.

Here, however, I was brought up standing. Sometimes the rods were more common in the head, sometimes in the thorax. I went at mosquito after mosquito spending hours over...

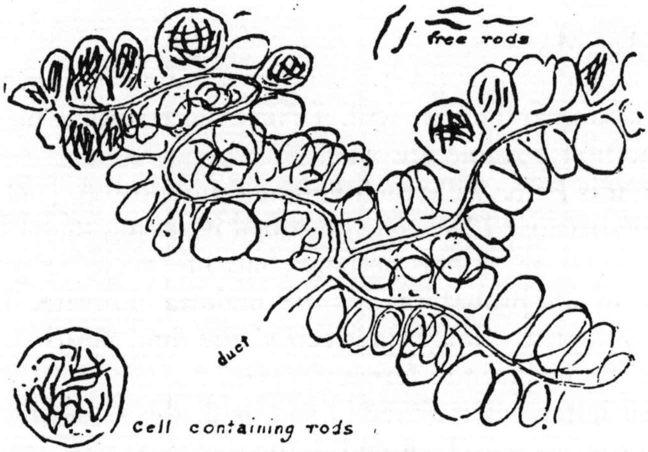

Germinal rods in salivary gland of mosquito. Published, from Ross's drawing, by Manson in *British Medical Journal*, 24 September 1898, page 852.[46]

[Unfortunately a part of the letter is here missing—probably sent to Lord Lister; but the missing part certainly described the following observation, recorded in my notes for 4 July for mosquito 22: "On taking up the thorax, which was first separated from the abdomen, a small round clear mass of tissue fell out and was seen to consist of mostly some worm-like gland with an air tube down the middle. Rods were very numerous here and were seen to be enclosed in numbers in clear cells attached to this gland (diagram)." The missing part of the letter probably contained the drawing above.]

...mosquitoes. In six of them the cells were packed (especially in some lobes) more or less with germinal rods. In the seventh I could find only a small piece of gland, which was free from rods.

I still experience, however, the greatest difficulty in dissecting out the gland itself. It appears to lie in front of the thorax close to the head but breaks so easily in the dissection that I cannot locate it properly. In the second mosquito, however, there was no doubt, as shown by evident attachment, that the duct led straight into the head-piece, probably into the mouth.

In other words it is a thousand to one it is a *salivary gland* [Plate I, fig 35].

I think that this, after further elaboration, will close at least one cycle of proteosoma and I feel that I am *almost* entitled to lay down the law by direct observation and tracking the parasite step by step—

Malaria is conveyed from a diseased person or bird to a healthy one by the proper species of mosquito and is inoculated by its bite.

Remember, however, that there is virtue in the "almost." I don't announce the law yet. Even when the microscope has done its utmost, healthy birds must be infected with all due precautions.

I say *one* cycle. I think it likely there is another. I continually observe that only a portion of the coccidia contain germinal rods. The rest, I now think, give rise to the black sausage-shaped bodies [Plate I, fig 34], which I believe may be the true spores of the parasite meant either for free life or to infect grubs. Oddly enough, in old mosquitoes these bodies also get carried away into the tissues—unless they are some disease of the insect. I will attack this next.

7th. I dissected two healthy mosquitoes this morning and began by dividing the head and anterior third of the thorax from the middle third by means of a razor and then carefully breaking up the anterior third. In both cases the glands were found and their ducts were traced straight into the head thus:

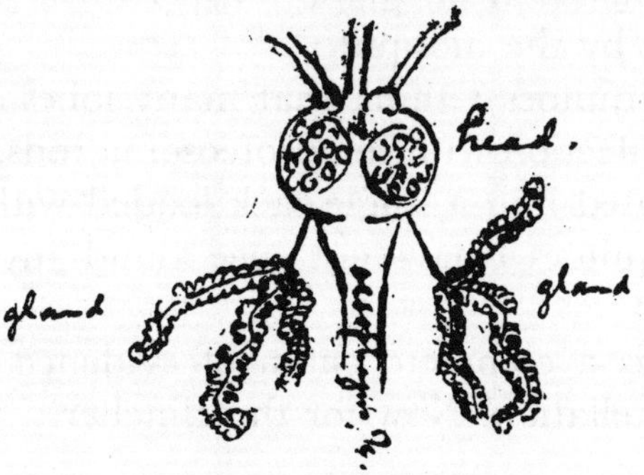

In all probability it is these glands which secrete the stinging fluid which the mosquito injects into the bite. The germinal rods lying, as they do, in the secreting cells of the gland pass into the duct when these cells begin to perform their function and are thus poured out in vast numbers under the skin of the man or bird. Arrived there, numbers of them are probably swept away by the circulation of the blood, in which they immediately begin to develop into malaria parasites, thus completing the cycle.

No time to write more.

Yours very sincerely,
R Ross.

Calcutta, 9 *July* 1898.

Dear Dr Manson,

One full solution of the malaria problem was obtained this morning—unfortunately just too late to catch the mail by wire to Bombay. The facts are as follows:

Just after I wrote to you I obtained some good dissections of the gland in healthy insects. It still remains very difficult to get out nicely and almost impossible to mount for you, but by examining a number of insects I have obtained the leading facts about it. The lobes lie either in the head, neck, or front of thorax (according to the fullness of the cells, I think), I think there are 18 lobes, thus [drawing—there are only six, as I soon found].

The ducts finally all join together into one large tube which runs up along the under surface of the head. In one specimen which I will send you I can trace it to its termination. When it arrives close to the orgin of the mouth parts it (the duct) passes through a kind of round shield and enters one of the long stabbing spears of the proboscis. It appears to run up *inside* this and open somewhere near its end.

There is no doubt then that the gland must pour its secretion straight into the wound made by the mosquito.

In old infected mosquitoes I think that many lobes of the gland are almost destroyed by infection with the proteosoma rods. In one case the cells seem to have united into a single sack loaded with rods.

In eight male mosquitoes I have not once found any evidence of the existence of this gland.

So far then there is a complete chain of evidence pointing to the infection during haustellation. Now for the clincher.

On the 25th June (as I think I told you) I carefully selected three healthy sparrows. Their blood had been examined three times on different occasions and always found free from parasites. On the 25th night and almost every night following I have used these birds to refeed a large stock of mosquitoes which had been infected from diseased sparrows on 21st–22nd June. This was the identical stock with which I worked out the story of the germinal rods. Lately I had been finding young crops of coccidia in this stock and therefore had a presentiment of what I should observe in the birds. I wish therefore I had examined them before so as to let you know in time for the BMA meeting but I hardly expected such a knock-down result.

All three birds, perfectly healthy a fortnight ago, were now simply swarming with proteosoma, 20 parasites and more in one oil-immersion field.

Again, on the 1st July I selected a healthy sparrow and a healthy "baia" and refed another infected stock on them every night up to date. These two were examined this morning. Both had proteosoma, the sparrow a few, the baia fairly numerous.

Hence I think I may now say QED and congratulate you on the mosquito theory indeed. The door is unlocked and I am walking in and collecting the treasures.

For instance, proteosoma of sparrows is communicable to baias. Hence there is probably only one proteosoma, common to various birds. You see, I shall give it to crows etc. Also, I have an idea indeed. What if proteosoma is spring tertian? I shall feed infected mosquitoes on a man or two and shall take it from a man to a sparrow if it be so.*

11th July. I have forgotten to say that 10 healthy sparrows examined on the 25th June and kept nightly in mosquito nets to keep mosquitoes *out* all remain perfectly well up to date. I told you also that on 25th June I gave infected mosquitoes to three healthy sparrows by the mouth. Two of the birds died a few days afterwards (numbers of my birds have been dying) without proteosoma. The third had nothing on 1st July and was used for feeding infected sparrows with positive results as already given. Rather a jumble, but future experiments will be more precise. It's useful to be jumbly at times to begin with.

I have now to record three more successes. Three baias (kind of bunting I think) were formerly found to contain large numbers of halteridium only—no proteosoma I am certain. They have often been

* Mahomed Bux, who had a bad attack of *P vivax* later on, thought he acquired it by being bitten by proteosoma infected mosquitoes.

used to refeed old infected stock. Yesterday they were examined again and found to contain numerous halteridium and *swarms* of proteosoma. One bird died last night. Liver enormous and black. Heart's blood contained an enormous young brood of proteosoma [drawing]. The bird's blood practically consisted of parasites. There you have it full at last. This also *proves* that sparrow's proteosoma is communicable to baias.

Having won the battle of Atbara I am now marching on to Omdurman—that is, I am rushing the black sausage-shaped bodies.... [I failed!]

Well, I have become unbearable with conceit over tracking the germinal rods into the salivary gland. That was a grand charge. I brag openly about it!...

The scheme you are going to propose is admirable. No doubt the Government of India will jog up when Chamberlain comes along. Remember I am entirely at your disposal. The idea is grand and I promise to throw myself into it. I have already arranged my tactics. They will be Napoleonic (!)—concentration. We shall attack one problem at a time in a body, if possible. That is the way, I am sure. See the results I am getting out of proteosoma alone....

... One single experiment with crescents (there are numerous dappled-winged mosquitoes here now) will enable me to bring human malaria into line with proteosoma—they are sure to be just the same. This will really score all the chief points. I ought to do it in two months; it has taken me only one to work out the germinal rod cycle....

I have had three and a half years' incessant work and worry, am feeling tired and out of sorts, and feel I should have a rest and get a sniff of cold before opening into such a big business as a commission....

... We are nearly ruined from having to live in hotels everywhere—family in one place, myself in another...

Yours sincerely,
R Ross.

CALCUTTA, 20 *July* 1898.

DEAR DR MANSON,

...Your letter to Harvey with Lord Lister's enclosure ought to do everything as to my being kept on at this work, but they won't give me assistance without pressure from the India Office. It is an excellent idea to send me a couple of men from a Colonial Office to learn the work. Last week I wrote asking to go home and I should certainly like to do so, but if you think it necessary will stay out longer in order to teach your men. *Do just as you like and think fit.*

Five more birds (sparrows) have been infected. Four healthy sparrows were bitten by old mosquitoes with germinal rods on the nights of the 10th–11th and 11th–12th July. They were examined again on the 18th. One was free (and died of tetanus same evening); the other three now swarmed with parasites, respectively two, six, and 10 in each field—proteosoma only of course.

On the 12th–13th and 13th–14th June five healthy sparrows were bitten by the same old stock (three weeks old). Two died next day and one on the 19th (no proteosoma). The remaining two had moderate proteosoma on the 18th day (sixth day of experiment).

Out of four control sparrows one showed a few proteosoma on the 7th day—probably overlooked before. The rest remain quite healthy.

I have calculated by calculus of probabilities the chances against birds becoming infected by accident *within a fortnight* after an experiment on the basis of the percentage of infected wild birds I have found. The chances are millions to one against three or four birds showing simultaneous accidental infection within the period. Apart from this, nine of the birds (I have infected 13) have had much more severe infections than I have ever seen before. I can therefore announce the law:

"Healthy birds may be infected by the bites of the proper species of mosquito which have previously fed on diseased birds."

I shall bring mathematics to bear heavily on these matters presently. Lucky I know something of the science (spent seven years over it). It will serve to knock on the head many loose ideas.

Not much work possible on the black bodies this week as I have been keeping my old stock for infecting sparrows. But I have failed to find the bodies in a large number of healthy mosquitoes so that I think they must be spores of the coccidia. They are carried by the circulation and distributed all over the tissues. The largest number of them seen by me in one insect is two or three hundred. A specimen kept for three weeks in the damp chamber shows no marked alteration or development of the bodies. They are too few to be meant to infect birds directly by the mouth or lungs. The chances would be infinity to one against one of them ever entering by these channels. What is a dead mosquito in water or dust? It is infinitesimal. Men and birds don't go about eating dead mosquitoes. No, Nature is too clever for such an attempt. She brings the mosquito (and the infection) straight to the man or bird and puts it nicely into his blood so as to give it every chance. I think then that the black bodies must be meant to infect grubs. They will probably produce germinal rods and infect the salivary glands again.

I am thinking of telegraphing to you, giving the result of the infection experiments. It may help you at the BMA....

Yours very sincerely,

R Ross.

CALCUTTA, 27 *July* 1898.

DEAR DR MANSON,

On the 25th, some more birds having become infected, particularly a crow, I made up my mind to wire to you announcing that one complete solution of the problem had been obtained. I think it may strengthen your hand at the BMA meeting and elsewhere and only wish I had done it before, as I might well have done.

On the same day yours of the 8th was received. It is dated the day before my first experimental batch of birds were found to be infected so that "following the spore into the bird" had been practically done when you wrote....

Much work has been doing. I forget how many birds have been announced to you as infected. Several fresh birds have come in, in spite of the fact that I have used very few mosquitoes. The only difference caused by doing this is that some of the birds (which were not bitten) escape. Those bitten have all very severe infections, quite exceeding what is ordinarily seen. The parasites begin to appear on the sixth, seventh, and eighth days and shortly reach vast numbers, five, 10, and more in a field when the bird dies. I found five young proteosoma in a single corpuscle.

I told you I would give sparrow's proteosoma to a crow. So I have. Parasites appeared first on the ninth day but have not become very numerous. They are utterly different from crow's halteridium and exactly like sparrow's proteosoma. These details must be left for future work and I am concentrating on the "black bodies."...

Yours sincerely,

R Ross.

Not only my "Report on the Cultivation of Proteosoma"[26] but also my letters, specimens, and telegram announcing the discovery of the "germinal threads" in the salivary glands of mosquitoes and the experimental infection of healthy birds by the bites of mosquitoes duly reached Manson before the meeting of the new tropical diseases section of the British Medical Association, which was held at Edinburgh on 26 to 29 July 1898. There, as president of the section, he gave a masterly account of his induction and of all my subsequent work up to the infection of birds as far as 25 July, when my telegram was sent.[46] This announcement was made less than six weeks after he had communicated the cultivation of proteosoma on 18 June[45] and, according to Dr Charles (page 212), it "created quite a furore." My friend Professor W J Simpson, who was present, has given me the following description of the event.

31 York Terrace,
York Gate, Regent's Park,
Nov 18, 1921.

My Dear Ross.

It was at the Edinburgh meeting of the British Medical Association in July of 1898 that Sir Patrick Manson was chairman of the tropical disease section. I attended all the meetings of this section and I remember the profound sensation produced among the members when Sir Patrick read out a telegram he had received from you describing your success in conveying malaria from bird to bird by means of "grey" mosquitoes fed on malaria-infected birds. At the same meeting were shown microscopical specimens which you had sent him demonstrating the progressive development of the malarial parasite in the mosquito. A resolution was unanimously passed sending you the members' congratulations on your great and epoch-making discovery.

I am glad to hear you are writing your memoirs.

With best wishes, believe me,

Yours sincerely,
W J Simpson.

Other distinguished men present were Dr William Osler of Baltimore and Professor Raphael Blanchard of Paris, the author of *Zoologie Médicale*, which had always been of so much use to me. The latter wrote me from Edinburgh on 28 July asking me for an article on my subject for his new *Archives de Parasitologie*, and adding, "*PS—M Manson a fait ce matin à la British Medical Association une communication du plus haut intéret sur vos recherches. Il me prie de vous presenter ses meilleurs compliments.*" The resolution of congratulation was proposed by Dr Andrew Davidson, of Edinburgh, the author of *Hygiene and Diseases of Warm Climates*, was seconded by Sir Joseph Ewart, and ran:

"That this section, recognising the great importance of the researches of Surgeon Major Ross on the development of the proteosoma in the mosquito in its bearings on the aetiology of human malaria, desires to convey to him through the president its deep sense of the obligations which all students of tropical pathology are under to this distinguished observer and to assure him of the interest and hope with which it follows his work."

The section also thanked Dr Manson "for having placed before the association the latest discoveries of Surgeon Major Ross with which his own name is so inseparably connected."

These details are given because someone was good enough to deny later that the meeting ever occurred! A full account of it, together with a copy of Plate I of my "Proteosoma report," was published in the first number of the new *Journal of Tropical Medicine*, edited by Dr James Cantlie (London), which appeared in August 1898; another, with one figure, in the *Lancet* of 20 August and an even fuller account, with several editorial notes, was given in the *British Medical Journal* for the 24 September 1898, together with the same plate and two other figures taken from the missing parts of my letters copied above which delineated the "germinal rods" by themselves and within the cells of the salivary gland. Appended to this last version, there is the following note:

"*Later Observations*

Note.—Letters received from Ross subsequently to the delivery of the foregoing confirm and expand what is therein stated. Many (30) successful experiments on the communication of proteosoma to healthy birds indicate an incubation period of from five to nine days. The intensity of the infection so conveyed gradually increases during several (four) days until finally as many as from five to ten or more parasites are to be found in every field of the bird's blood. These artificial infections are much more severe than those acquired naturally; the birds may die from them." [The note goes on to record my observations supporting Mannaberg's view that the sexual forms may be produced by conjugation and my studies of the black spores.]

Manson was doubtful whether malaria is communicated only by the bite of the mosquito for he said:

That this is the last word on the subject of the extracorporeal phase of the malaria parasite I do not believe. I think that malaria may be acquired in this way—that is, by the bite of the mosquito—but that that is the only way I cannot venture to assert, in fact I do not think. For observe; malaria, we know, multiplies indefinitely outside the human body, independently of man. In fact, malaria is most prevalent in places where man is not.* Therefore this extracorporeal condition of multiplication must demand something more than a short cycle of from man to mosquito and from mosquito to man. My impression is that it requires an infection of mosquito by mosquito; possibly, as in tick disease or as in silk worm disease through the insect's ova, possibly through the larva. Ross's facts supply us, gentlemen, with an explanation of the former sort. They do not tell us how the parasite multiplies indefinitely through generation after generation. Still, it is a most important addition to our knowledge and I am sure that it will lead to a full solution of the entire problem and to very many advances in this important subject. It may be objected that what holds good for proteosoma may not hold good for *Plasmodium malariae*. But the similarity of the parasites is so great that one cannot resist the conclusion that their histories are also similar. Moreover, Ross has distinctly shown, as already mentioned, that certain species of mosquito do elaborate pigmented cells when fed on human malarial blood.

"I am sure that you will agree with me that the medical world, I might even say humanity, is extremely indebted to Surgeon Major Ross for what he has already done and I am sure you will agree with me that every encouragement and assistance should be given to so hard working, so intelligent, and so successful an investigator to continue his work."

As shown in my letter to him of 20 July, I was not exactly of this opinion: I thought that Nature "brings the mosquito (and the infection) straight to the man or bird and puts it nicely into his blood" and that this was the only way in which *men and birds* became infected, but I also thought that the "black spores" possibly infect *mosquito grubs* from their parents, which may have died in the water in which they laid their eggs, thus carrying on the infection from mosquito to mosquito independently of men or birds. But this was only a speculation requiring experimental

* I showed later, especially in another publication,[47] that there has never been any real evidence for this statement.

proof and in the meantime the fact remained that malaria was carried from man to mosquito and from mosquito to man.

Thus the great victory was won at last. It gave us simultaneously two important advances in knowledge.

Zoologically, the case of *Proteosoma relicta* was the first one in which the great law of metaxeny of alternation of host (page 8) was proved to apply to unicellular parasites as it had been known for years to apply to higher parasites; and it was certain by zoological homology to occur (though possibly with some small modifications) in other members of the same group, including the three species of malaria parasite of men and also, very probably, in some other unicellular parasites.

From the *epidemiological* point of view the discovery showed us that the malaria infection is not acquired from drinking water nor from the inhalation of marsh air or "miasmata" but is put directly into our blood by the bite of mosquitoes. King had thought of this in 1883 (page 10); Manson had not supported the idea; I had considered it possible (page 72); but none of us had really even imagined the wonderful process which had now been discovered on 4 and 9 July. Nature was more resourceful and astute than all of us. She did not spill the germs broadcast through the soil, water, and air, as we had supposed; she put them directly into man from the mosquito and into the mosquito from man! And this would render more instant and exact the means of preventing the greatest of diseases.

Apart from such considerations, the entry of the "germinal threads" into the veneno-salivary glands of the mosquito is surely, perhaps, the most wonderful and beautiful case of natural design which we know of—difficult to explain by evolution even today.

I will not attempt to describe my feelings to the reader—especially as he may already be weary of such excursions. Then indeed—

> Then felt I like some watcher of the skies
> When a new planet swims into his ken.

Such moments come only to one or two persons in a generation. The pleasure is greater than that given by any triumph of the orator, the statesman, or the conqueror; for the end attained does not lie in some petty intertribal advantage but in a benefit conferred upon all men and not only for today but for all time—at least until "the future dares forget the past." The triumph of 20 August 1897 was now completed and crowned by that of 9 July 1898—more than enough to compensate me for all my toils.

But now Dame Fortune, who had conferred such a great bounty upon me, tightened her lips and her purse strings and did nothing but buffet me for the remainder of my time in India! First she sent me the "black spores" to worry me for weeks. Then she gave me the dapple-winged mosquito, *Anopheles rossi*, which does not carry malaria at all. She continued the plague scare. She made the Royal Society refuse to send me help. She instigated Surgeon General Harvey to interrupt my work for months on the kala-azar inquiry. And lastly she arranged that some ingenious Italian gentlemen should pirate most of my results in the interval. "*Souvent femme varie/Bien fol est qui s'y fie!*"

The *black spores* were first discovered by me, appropriately enough, on 1 April—large, brown, sausage-shaped objects. As they occurred in clusters actually within the ripe proteosoma coccidia and (at first) only in infected mosquitoes it was natural to infer that they might constitute a developmental stage of the parasites; and as it was my first duty to work out thoroughly the whole life cycle of proteosoma before beginning more showy work on the human plasmodia I was obliged to expend much valuable time and labour on the subject. I tried to infect birds and mosquito larvae with them—in vain; and it was not until January 1899 that I found them in uninfected mosquitoes and began to be convinced (I had already suspected it, page 171) that they were only parasites within parasites. They are now thought to belong to the genus Nosema. One of my quasiscientific friends later accused me of being "deluded" by these bodies, but I was quite right to investigate them thoroughly.

The *Anopheles rossi* were large dapple-winged mosquitoes not unlike those in which I had first found the pigmented cells in Secunderabad in 1897 and also like those I saw in Oodeypur. They began to appear in my laboratory about this time, but I was still not allowed to work with human malaria there owing to the plague scare. My men, however, found their larvae—in water on *the ground.*

Some few more extracts from letters to Manson. On the 3rd August I wrote:

"The black spores refuse to capitulate; the result is that I am nearly dead with work again. They *don't* change in water or in dead mosquitoes, though kept—for periods ranging to six weeks nearly. They *don't* change in the stomach of medium and large grubs. By feeding these on torn-up mosquitoes with black spores I can get as many as I like (as many as 500) of the latter into their stomachs—but not a sign of change. I am now trying very young grubs and have also fed five healthy sparrows with the spores.

"Numerous most beautiful demonstrations of the germinal rods (what *shall* we call them?) in the salivary glands, but fixed specimens almost impossible to make. Also some very good specimens of coccidia of 10th day breaking up into black spores.... I am dying to finish proteosoma as I am beginning to knock up more than ever. Nothing but work as hard as I can go for two months. Am beginning to be sleepless. (Illegible) fear all the same, as you may imagine but most trying to eyes and brain.

"As you say, proteosoma should be finished and then the human germs can easily be tackled. Unfortunately that kala-azar weighs on me like a nightmare. I do hope you will be all right when this reaches you."

On 11 August I wrote:

"I have not much to tell you this week. Three out of five birds fed with seven infected mosquitoes each on the 31st—many of the mosquitoes containing black spores—have all remained healthy to date, while several birds bitten on 3rd to 4th night were attacked the day before yesterday. Apparently no outlet here. I have fed many grubs of all sizes on the spores. Crowds of the spores in their stomach tube, but they are passed out and found in the droppings quite unchanged. Spores in the damp chamber remain the same.

"I fancy some condition of ripening is required. This obtained, I fancy the spores will infect the grubs, grow into coccidia, and give rise to germinal rods and spores again. Well, I am dead beat and have asked leave to go to Kurseong for a few weeks *en route* for Assam. I have lost 11 pounds in weight the last two months. Work at the microscope all night, can't sleep, and feel as low as possible."

My next letter was from Kurseong, 23 August 1898:

"I had to leave Calcutta abruptly on the 13th, much specimen-making and photo-taking incomplete. I had practically ceased to sleep—worked at microscope all night—and began to forget everything. Since coming here I have thought it best not to think of the germs at all. When I am in work I go too hard at it and can't shake it off my mind with the result that I knock up in a month or two, especially in a hot climate. However, the hard part of the work is over.

"I fear that you also overdid it a great deal for your health at the BMA meeting. Many thanks for your letters up to the 5th August and for copy of the resolution of the tropical section, which is indeed flattering! I rather think, however, that they put the two paragraphs in the wrong order! The idea is of the first importance; the brain is over the hand. My function in this work has only been of the hand—that is a point I stick to. You would have polished off the whole matter in a quarter of the time I have taken. When the time comes to write the history of the whole campaign—it will have to be a separate book, not an article, I think—this will be brought into full relief, I promise you."*

This letter concluded with a four-page summary of my results from 4 June to 31 August 1898, including details of the infection experiments.[49,50]

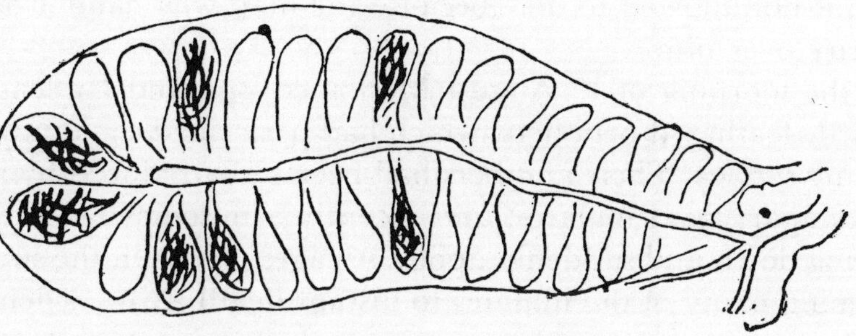

Germinal rods in salivary gland of mosquito. From letter of Ross to Laveran, 18 July 1898.

I sent similar summaries to Laveran. During my stay in India I wrote him seven letters containing 29 pages, dated 12 February 1896, 23 January, 25 April, 18 July, 2 September, 15 November 1898, and 3 January 1899. Those of April and July 1898 gave him all the facts about proteosoma in mosquitoes, with drawings of the germinal rods in the salivary gland, and the infection of healthy birds.

On 2 September 1898 I wrote:

"It is worthy to note that the grey mosquitoes which are the definitive hosts of proteosoma breed in pots, barrels, and ditches containing water, even at a height of 6000 feet (2000 metres) above the sea. On the contrary, the dappled-winged mosquitoes which I believe carry paludism breed only in small puddles of rainwater where there are no fish or frogs which eat them. These facts seem to explain the telluric and meteorologic conditions of these forms of parasitism.... "

Years later Laveran lent me the original letters to have copies made—which I now possess.

I left Calcutta with a heavy heart for the wretched kala-azar duty. The great treasurehouse had been opened, but I was dragged away before I could handle the treasures. Scores of beautiful researches now lay open to me. I should have followed the "vermicule" in the

* There are many prophets in Israel—but very few disciples!

mosquito's stomach—that was left to Robert Koch. I intended to mix the "germinal threads" with birds' blood—that was left to Schaudinn. I wished to complete the cycle of the human parasites—that was left to the Italians and others. I had designed numerous experiments on immunity in malaria and on the treatment of the disease—most of which have never been done even yet. The last mentioned research alone might have saved Britain millions of pounds during the war. No, the man who can do is not allowed to do—because the man who cannot do is put in authority over him.

On the morning of 13 August Mahomed Bux and I released all our poor little feathered prisoners, which had performed such unwitting and unwilling service. Their numbers had been sadly reduced by mysterious illnesses apart from malaria, and recently a mischievous hawk took to swooping down and suddenly upon the cages placed in the sunshine and frightening many of the inmates to instant death. Now, when the doors of the cages were opened many refused to go out and others even returned after going out. Some were weak and ill, but finally we got them all safely into the trees and bushes after driving away cats and firing a shot at the hawk. May their little souls be living for ever among eternal flowers and berries in some avian heaven. Mahomed, who had given names to most of them, looked almost sad as they departed.

10

The Third Interruption. Assam, 1898

As I have stated, one object of this book is to give the lay reader a real picture of that rather rare thing, a real medical investigation and of its consequences. I will therefore beg him to consider the following question: What should our nation have done in response to that memorable announcement of Manson's at the British Medical Association meeting in July 1898? If, let us say, a geological prospector had discovered gold or diamonds or oil somewhere in India then there would have been an immediate stir; hundreds of people would have flocked to him and the authorities would have been forced to notice and regulate the subsequent work. Or if, let us say, a hill tribe had committed some depredation the authorities would have brought up an army against them at the cost of millions of rupees. But what was the situation now regarding malaria? It has been estimated to cause (the reader is doubtless weary of hearing it!) about 1 300 000 deaths every year in India alone, not to mention an enormous amount of sickness—almost equal to the mortality caused by the Great War; it was incommoding or paralysing most of the planting industries in India and was, perhaps, the principal cause of unnecessary expense during all military expeditions. Now a solitary worker in India had suddenly revolutionised our knowlege (or rather ignorance) of it by showing exactly how it is communicated to us. What—unless we were to be admitted a race of unintellectual slugs—should the British authorities everywhere have done to meet this new situation? They should have sent immediately to that solitary worker not one but a dozen assistants, medical men, biologists, entomologists, besides subordinates to learn his technique, to classify mosquitoes, to ascertain which of them carry the three species of human malaria, to study their habits, to determine how best, with the new knowledge, the disease may be prevented on the large scale, and *to prevent it*. Not only should the Indian Government have allotted a handsome credit for this work, but every malarious colony in the Empire should have joined and the work should have been commenced throughout our domininions, at least, within a year. What actually happened? My work was not assisted but interrupted for five whole months; one doctor was sent to me afterwards for a few weeks at the worst possible season to inquire whether I had been speaking the truth; I was forced to retire after six months because I could obtain no definite assurance that I was to be continued at the work; and now, 23 years after the event, probably not one tithe of the programme sketched above has been carried out within the British Empire! It will be instructive to give the details—and possibly amusing.

As soon as the mosquito theory was proved in March–April 1898 both Manson and I saw that immediate assistance was required—vide my letters of 16 and 30 May (pages 159, 161). Mr Joseph Chamberlain was then Secretary of State at the Colonial Office, Manson being its medical adviser, and Lord Lister was president of the Royal Society. On 6 June, probably after receiving my letter of 16 May, Manson wrote:

"I went to see Lord Lister yesterday. He promised to go over your work and give his opinion upon it, to say whether he thought it of sufficient public importance to go with to Government and tell them they must go on with it. A week ago I saw Chamberlain, who wants investigations made on the African fevers and who is willing to make a grant for this purpose. I told Chamberlain that important investigations were in progress in India which were about to be made public and asked him to wait for a week or two to get Lord Lister's expression of opinion on their value before going to the Treasury for the money.... I will suggest a commission with you at the head of it and will get Lister to back me up.... PS Lister was very sympathetic and encouraging."

On 24 June Manson wrote:

"On Tuesday I got Lister to come to my house and had some six or seven microscopes with your preparations for him to study. I was very ill at the time but struggled with clothes and told him all about the matter. He expressed himself convinced. I asked him if he would back me up in my representation to the government. He said he would and was everything you could desire in his recognition of the value of your discovery.... I shall suggest that the Colonial Government either make a grant for the continuation of the investigation or (agree) to send over two men to be under and assist you and so qualify for working out the problem in Africa and other colonies. I shall say that time, a free hand, and adequate finances are necessary.... A permanent commission appointed with yourself at the head."

With his next letter of 1 July Manson enclosed a copy of the following open one from Lord Lister:

12 Park Crescent, Portland Place,
29 *June* 1898.

Dear Dr Manson,

I return the copy of Dr Ross's report with best thanks for the opportunity of reading it.

Taken in conjunction with the preparations which you kindly showed me it seems to me to be of remarkable interest and value and I regard it as most desirable that his experience and, I may add, his manipulative skill should be turned to further account by opportunity being given him of continuing his researches on the subject.

Very sincerely yours,
Lister.

On 8 July Manson wrote again:

"I think things are going on well on this side. Mr Chamberlain has written to Lord Lister to the effect that he wants something done in the malaria line and saying that the Colonial Government will bear half the expense. Lister called on me yesterday and I posted him again on the mosquito business so that he might be ready for the committee meeting of the Royal Society yesterday afternoon which was to discuss Chamberlain's letter. I suggested two medical men and an entomologist to go to India to help and learn from you, who might afterwards be sent to Africa or elsewhere to take up the inquiry. I think it will be all right now. At all events the Indian Government will see that whatever they think about the matter it is considered one of the first importance here."

Manson's scheme was admirable, especially because he hoped that the Indian authorities would thus be persuaded to place additional assistants under me for purely Indian work. I heard nothing further about the matter for a month, but on 5 August Manson wrote: "The Royal Society proposals are not good—at all events to my mind. They want to send a research scholar to you and two bacteriologists, I suppose to study blackwater fever in Central Africa. This is quite inadequate and I went expressly to the Colonial Office to say so. The enclosed I have just received and I shall have another try for a full commission on the original line I suggested. I hope I may succeed. Your discovery is either the most important of the *fin de siècle* or it is nothing. I shall do all I can for it on the first assumption and try to make England work it." The enclosure referred to was a request that Manson should meet Chamberlain and Lister next day. On 9 August he wrote: "The Royal Society wished to send two biologists to Africa to study malaria. They said medical men knew nothing of biology." Finally it came to this, that Dr C W Daniels, of Demerara, was nominated by Manson to come out to me and that the rest of my "commission" evaporated into thin air or, what was the same thing, into Africa to study blackwater fever.

In my experience almost any and every committee, even of the cleverest men, is sure to make a mess of almost any and every business entrusted to it if it can possibly do so, and this committee paralysed malaria work in India for years. I do not know, and do not wish to know, who composed it—probably some worthy English doctors and zoologists not one of whom had made a special study of malaria or of its parasites, or knew of my difficulties, or grasped exactly what it was we wanted. Manson, who was not then a fellow of the Royal Society, seems never to have been asked to attend its weighty deliberations. Afterwards I heard that it was turned against me by two supreme faults in my "Report on the Cultivation of Proteosoma."[26] One was that the shading in two of my drawings was hurriedly scribbled with the pen instead of being etched in parallel lines and the other was that zoological names were not printed in italics. I hope the people of India will forgive these people some day—certainly I will never do so! Evidently the case of Galilei and the scholastics of Pisa over again.

So I was to have no assistance, but the Director General might at least have allowed me to finish the malaria work single-handed. As already stated (page 162), I wrote to him direct on 25 May urging that it would be impossible to combine that work with such a difficult task as the kala-azar investigation. His secretary replied on 2 June that malaria should have precedence over kala-azar, but I was not excused the latter duty and assistance was refused; and my special duty was to conclude on 17 August. There was, however, a simple way out of the difficulty. My first small pension was due to me in June and I could apply at once to be allowed to take it as soon as my malaria duty was to end. This would have enabled me to avoid wasting my time over kala-azar, and I even proposed to go to Italy in order to continue the malaria work there unhampered on my way home. Such would indeed have been much the best course, if only to bring matters to a head, and I was on the point of sending in my papers in June when Manson's scheme of the commission reached me. After that, as I did not like to disappoint him, I applied on 1 July for six months' extension of the special duty. It was granted on 18 July. Meantime on 9 July I reported the infection of healthy birds and again hinted at being excused the kala-azar duty. On the 13th Surgeon Major Leslie replied from Simla: "The DG desires me to say how much he is interested and how pleased he is with the success which is being obtained by you in your investigations." That was all. Nothing about being excused kala-azar. So I was doomed! For the second time I was to be interrupted just as I had the conclusion of the human malaria work within easy reach. Already much wearied with the old task, I was to undertake a new and utterly different one which would occupy me for months. Columbus, having sighted America, was ordered off to discover the North Pole! I left Calcutta on 13 August and a week later heard that Manson's scheme for a commission had collapsed.

The reader will not be long detained over kala-azar. It is a fever, not intermittent like malaria, but one which continues for months with long waves of improvement or exacerbation during which the spleen and usually the liver become enormously enlarged and the patient thins to a living skeleton—somewhat like ankylostomiasis (hookworm disease) on the one hand and chronic malaria on the other. But the malady was worse than either: whole families, villages, and coolies' quarters were affected and it was a dreadful sight to see the poor wretches, nothing but skin and bone, with enormous abdomens, children and adults, trying to keep alive by lying in the sunshine—and death was then almost inevitable. It is sights like these which make the medical investigator.

Kala-azar (black sickness) was first mentioned in the *Annual Sanitary Report for Assam*, written by Dr Clarke, for 1881, page 28; and in the similar report for 1882 a description of the disease is given, based on a report by Mr McNaught,* then civil medical officer at Tura, Garo Hills, Assam, who studied 120 cases of the disease and the epidemiology of it, and who discovered the malady. As it spread in Assam most of the medical officers thought it was only a very virulent form of malaria, but

* I believe that Mr McNaught was then only an assistant surgeon. He was given commissioned rank later and was a Captain IMS at Nowgong when I was there. I cannot find his name in Colonel D G Crawford's *History of the Indian Medical Service* (London, 1914) and he seems never to have received any acknowledgement for his most important discovery.

others doubted this and in November 1889 Surgeon Major G M Giles, IMS, was put on special duty to report upon it. He concluded that it was hookworm disease, but as the local medical officers resisted this opinion also the Government sent Surgeon Captain Leonard Rogers, IMS, in April 1896 to make further investigations and he concluded that it was malaria. I was now required in 1898 to decide and ended by supporting Rogers (with some amendments). We were all wrong. The disease is one of another class which exists in many parts of the world, Old and New, causes many kinds of illness, and is due to various species of a new genus of parasite called by me in 1903 Leishmania.[51] The difficulty of my task may be gauged from the fact that most cases of kala-azar are *also* heavily infected both with hookworms and with malaria, being cases of what I called herodiasis or multiple parasitism, and that at that time we did not generally use in India the Romanowsky method of staining, which is almost essential for distinguishing the leishmania. Even Manson scarcely recommended it in the first edition of his *Tropical Disease*, 1898, page 31. I *ought* to have used it; if I had done so I should doubtless have found the leishmania myself, besides being able to stain my "proteosoma coccidia" and "germinal threads" better than I had done; but I had really had not time to study new staining methods while in the midst of making my fundamental "differential experiments."

Just as I was about to leave Calcutta for Assam I heard that Captain E Harold Brown, MD, IMS, had recently been investigating an allied disease of Bengal called kala-dukh (black or deadly pain) and that there was a similar sickness in the Darjeeling Terai called either kala-dukh or kala-jwar (black fever). The latter area was close to Kerseong, where my wife and family still were, and I obtained permission to go there first. Leaving Calcutta on 13 August 1898, wearied out with heat and work, I spent a few days at Kurseong doing some odd jobs and on the 24th proceeded with Mahomed Bux and Lutchman to a place called Naxalbari, about nine miles out on the plain, supposed to be the centre of kala-jwar. We lived there with some very kind planters (Mr Longmore and friends) who, like Horace, scorned mosquito nets and had constant fever but who solaced themselves by playing beautifully on the violin! About this visit I wrote:

KURSEONG, 6 *September* 1898.

DEAR DR MANSON,

I spent a week at Naxalbari. Results poor. In about 100 persons examined malaria parasites were found only in five or six, though numbers of the cases had enormous spleens with a kind of hectic fever. The cases were evidently old malarial infections. As the people always refused to stay for repeated examinations motions could not be often looked at for eggs. Not a single suitable case for mosquito feedings was obtained.

The mosquitoes were dappled-wings and greys. The former breed in rain puddles exclusively I think. Hence the whole climatic variations of aestivoautumnal. I examined numbers of both kinds caught in houses of fever cases. No coccidia or rods. As, however, the fever cases in question had only a few wretched young parasites in a whole specimen, infection of mosquitoes was unlikely. I did not see a single crescent the whole time (remember what Rogers said). No rods were seen in the salivary glands of many mosquitoes. The dapple-wings bite very fiercely. Their grubs float horizontally like sticks in the puddles, a noteworthy and very useful peculiarity.

I don't believe that fresh malaria was about at all at Naxalbari at this season. There were floods of rain which continually scoured out the puddles. People said that there were very few mosquitoes. Dapple-wings won't live in any but the smallest puddles because the minnows which swarm in anything over a few gallons' capacity devour them instantly. Malaria is probably a *very* easily prevented disease. I preached mosquito nets and antipuddle propaganda and left. Tomorrow I am off to Assam....

The real Terai disease is probably ankylostomiasis and not malaria. Many frightful cases of the former. Hospital assistant at Naxalbari had never *heard* of it! The worst cases of mere malaria with spleens touching livers looked quite cheerful and jolly.

Filaria is also present you will be *glad* to hear. I made the following most interesting observations which you may like to add to your filaria lore. While examining mosquitoes I took some grey ones caught in a mosquito net within which a native catechist, his wife, and one child, all with fever, slept nightly. The thorax was seen to contain something new. It was a development stage of fsh.* Numerous forms of all stages up to the full active stage were easily found in all of five mosquitoes examined. Evidently our catechist was too lazy to kill his mosquito in the morning. Taking his night blood I found *F nocturna*. A case of filaria diagnosed through the mosquito!—and a very easy way of diagnosing it too. I shall employ it clinically some day.

* *Filaria sanguinis hominis.*

Have had a great disappointment. P D Simond* has been here. I wrote and he came down to see me. I had just gone to Naxalbari. He followed me down the line but it was no use, he had to be in Calcutta on a fixed date and we did not meet after all. I would have given much to have shown him the work and found out something about coccidia.

I have had a nice letter from Nuttall.†

Have written officially to Government and asked for permission to publish. The present state of things is very annoying.

I thought you would not find the Royal Society rise easily to your fly.... I shall be in Assam in a few days. Don't expect to be able to do anything at all with kala-azar at this season. All the malaria cases will be probably stale ones—no parasites—nothing decisive. But I shall make every effort to bring at least one of the human parasites into line with proteosoma. (Am very apprehensive about not finding crescents.) This done (with luck it may be done in a week or two), if kala-azar turns out unfruitful I may come back to Calcutta by 1st November, where I can demonstrate to Daniels and the other man....

I see by the *BMJ* for August 20th, p 498, that Koch has gone to Italy to study malaria. It is quite possible that he will at once succeed in infecting men by the mosquito if he is lucky. In the meantime I am absolutely forbidden to publish anything about my infection of birds....

Yours sincerely,
R Ross.

The first part of this letter indicates my malaria doctrine at the time, including the attitude of anopheline larvae, their breeding habits, their destruction by fish, and the prevention of malaria by protection and mosquito reduction—all of which have been frequently discovered since then quite *indipendentemente da Ross* of course! I find from my notebook that altogether 10‡ dapple-winged mosquitoes (caught in one of Mr Longmore's godowns in which there was a sick servant) were examined on that occasion. By bad luck all were negative. They were mostly *Anopheles listoni*, in which Stephens and Christophers, with better fortune, easily found zygotes later in this very district.

Leaving Kurseong on 9 September I travelled by train and steam

* Of the Pasteur Institute, who had written on the flagellate forms of the *Coccidium oviforme* of rabbits, page 130.

† See page 208.

‡ This is the correct number. I said "some dozens" in my Nobel Lecture.

ferries to the bank of the Brahmaputra near Jatrapur, whence we took the river steamer on 10 September. The great river was in flood—not in a trench between steep banks like the Irrawaddy but a vast islanded expanse of swirling brown water up which the steamer panted slowly. We (Mahomed, Lutchman, and myself) reached Gauhati in Assam on the 11th and, after seeing some cases there, arrived at Nowgong on the 13th. This I described to my wife as "not at all a bad little place. A pretty full-fed river winds along in front of the station, which is built on flat ground with large trees between the houses ... will you send me my fishing things?" It was now the centre of kala-azar, which had moved hither from the Garo Hills, and Dr McNaught himself was in charge of the hospital. I lived most of the time with Mr W J Reid, ICS, the district magistrate—an able young officer who was extremely kind to me and helped me in every possible way. I remained there examining numbers of cases, doing postmortems, and taking depositions until 21 October, after which I moved, with Reid, to Mr G Jamieson's bungalow not far away. This was the place where a tiger had walked in one night and taken out a planter by the hand (between his teeth) in order to eat him fresh outside!—the planter was rescued but his hair had turned white! Thence I went to Umluki, Silghat, and Tezpur in order to take the depositions of Drs Lavertine, Dodds-Price, and Macnamara, all men of great experience with regard to kala-azar. On 26 October we took boat again at Gauhati and on the 28th reached Kurseong again, where I commenced my report on kala-azar.

Apparently the reason why Giles considered kala-azar to be hookworm disease was that he never met McNaught and was presumably never shown true cases of kala-azar. Directly I arrived at Nowgong and was shown cases by McNaught I concluded at once that they were not hookworm disease and told Manson so in my letter of 9 October. The only question now was whether kala-azar was merely malaria or something quite different. The early stages were indistinguishable by me then; and no wonder, because most of them had the double infection. But later the kala-azar cases showed an enormous enlargement of the spleen and liver with continued fever, which were, at best, not common in simple malaria. On pricking these organs in living patients at this stage and also in half a dozen necropsies I seldom found malaria parasites or pigment and hence might have rightly but rashly concluded at once that they were not malaria. Indeed this was my opinion for some weeks. But there was another possible explanation of this absence. The cases may have been originally due only to severe malaria which had gradually died out of them owing to the establishment of personal immunity, leaving them wrecks with permanently damaged spleen and liver. How could this happen? The medical dogma of the time was that there was no immunity in or against malaria, but I saw at once, as the logical result of my findings in July, that there must be immunity in malaria (quite apart from the kala-azar question). I think this was first announced by me in my letter to Manson of 16 October from Nowgong:

"Now why does the parasitic invasion cease after a time? Certainly not in consequence of quinine because these people don't take it. This is my theory. *Immunity* is established. Compare my results with the reinfection of sparrows. Probably these kala-azar cases become infected over and over again in the early stages by mosquitoes which have bitten themselves previously—or their diseased relatives—and they would simply perish straight off unless some process of immunity were established. This is established, but the organs are left wrecked.

"Hence kala-azar at the stage when it is usually diagnosed as such is in reality no longer a haemamoebiasis curable by quinine but a kind of spleen and liver disease with the *fièvre symptomatique* of Kelsch and Kiener and yellow pigment only. The main incidence falls on the liver.

"The main point to fix the mind on is that in these severe untreated cases of malaria a species of immunity is established in a few months, which enables the system to eliminate the parasites itself but only at the expense of profound siderosis and often ultimate destruction of the liver and in a less degree of the spleen. Compare Kelsch and Kiener's cases of 'Chronic malaria.'

"Among Europeans who treat themselves with quinine and are not nearly so exposed to mosquito infection and reinfection this immunity is seldom established so that they frequently have attacks of haemamoebic fever to the last, giving, of course, the usual black pigmentation."

Again, on 15 November, I wrote to him from Kurseong: "My solution is that immunity against the parasites is established after a month or two, after which the black pigment is eliminated but the pathological condition of the organs (due possibly to the yellow pigment) remains. The disease must be malaria as every gradation from early cases with parasites and (black) pigment in the spleen to established kala-azar cases without either existed." Nevertheless I was wrong! But the theory of immunity here indicated still holds for malaria in general.

It was another medical dogma of the time that the black malarial pigment is never eliminated when once deposited in certain organs. This had been completely disproved by my recent observations on birds: more pigment was often found in a bird which had been infected only for a few days than in one which had been equally heavily infected for a month.

When Rogers said that kala-azar was malaria he was disbelieved because of a third medical dogma, that malaria is not communicated from man to man as kala-azar is. This, of course, had also been disposed of by my results of July.

When I was sent on this wild-goose chase neither myself nor, I believe, the Director General ever dreamed that, apart from the investigation itself, the actual writing of the report would occupy me for months; but this was the case. The necessity of discussing all these points, of examining innumerable pathological details, of consulting authorities (none too sound), and of reconsidering the subject with Dr C W Daniels (who arrived before Christmas) compelled me to waste upon it nearly the whole of my time from the end of October to the end of January 1899. The report[52] covers nearly 90 foolscap pages of close print. I was tired when I commenced it, gradually became so fatigued that I could scarcely write a page a day, and ended by being utterly "fagged out" by it. Yet all this precious time and labour might have been spent on finding the carriers of the human plasmodia and in finishing, describing, and figuring properly my work done in July and August, my observations on mosquitoes, and my full technique.

Of course, owing to the press of pathological work, serious mosquito work was impossible at Nowgong, but I fed 15 dapple-wings (*mostly A rossi*) and 11 elephant mosquitoes (*Panoplites sp*) on a case with a few crescents and on another with quartan malaria. All were negative, but the feeding was left to assistants. I also examined a few insects caught in the houses of patients.*

During my stay at Nowgong I wrote for Government a short "Preliminary Report on the Infection of Birds with Proteosoma by the Bites of Mosquitoes."[49] It gave little more information than Manson gave at the British Medical Association meeting in July.[46]

I think I saw the leishmania several times in the small quantities of spleen pulp which I often extracted from patients by means of a hypodermic syringe—on payment of a *douceur* of two or three annas; but I cannot be sure because the stain was not used. This little operation,

* Nowgong was full of panoplites with their extraordinary egg, like a kind of tobacco pipe. I first saw and figured these in Calcutta on 31 March 1898 (page 152) and afterwards showed both eggs and mosquitoes to C W Daniels.

which was almost painless and quite harmless, was often the source of some amusement because after a time the children almost demanded it. One boy called Pual said it made him feel so much better; perhaps this was due to the sweets which he bought with the money!

On 18 November we all left beautiful Kurseong for Calcutta, where we had been obliged to take an expensive flat at 31 Chowringee. After entering it we soon discovered that empty tin packing cases were being hammered into shape all day long in the back yard of a neighbouring shop—good for writing my report! My laboratory was ready for me, but alas! I had no time to use it. There we remained until my period of special duty terminated (16 February 1899) and we left India for good.

I see by my notebook that we started work again to some small extent on 25 November. But the conditions had now changed: comparatively few of the wild birds were infected and the mosquitoes refused to bite in the dry cool air of that season in Calcutta. We had some old incubators in the laboratory, but the smell of the gas, or something else, offended our fastidious victims.

During all my stay in Calcutta scarcely anyone except Dr Dyson, IMS, the deputy sanitary commissioner, and Dr Cooke, the health officer, had ever troubled to see my work, though the city was full of doctors and professors. But in October, when I was in Assam Dr S W Rivenburg, of the American Mission there, wrote and asked permission to join me in Calcutta. He was quite unknown to me but arrived with his wife and children (at his own expense) on about the 26 November. Of course he came to learn; but he also helped and I respected him much for his enterprise.

On 22 December the long-expected succour from the Royal Society arrived at last in the shape of Dr C W Daniels, of British Guiana. I had particularly wanted an entomologist to classify my mosquitoes, but Daniels was not one and, moreover, could not help me with the Romanowsky stain. He had, however, a great experience of malaria, a knowledge of its pathology, and a sound scientific judgment (short of mathematics); and he assisted me greatly in preparing my kala-azar report. On arrival he was polite but cold and evidently sceptical even of my old proteosoma results. In fact he had not been sent to assist me but first to ascertain whether I had been speaking the truth and secondly, if so, to "suck" my brains! The unfortunate committee which sent him might have saved itself the expense because dozens of specimens proving my case were in Manson's hands in London at the time and my technique had already been sufficiently described in my "Report on the Cultivation of Proteosoma." But nevertheless we welcomed him and he was soon convinced. Later on he and Rivenburg succeeded in infecting 12 out of 22 healthy sparrows by the bites of *Culex fatigans*; but though we at last procured two good cases of crescents and used incubators, we failed to infect any dapple-wings. There were two reasons for this: most of these mosquitoes were *Anopheles rossi* Giles, now known to be negative to malaria, and secondly the nights were cold and we had no warm chamber. For this latter reason the transmission experiments of proteosoma also often failed, the pigmented cells developed much more slowly, and a much smaller proportion of wild sparrows were found infected. Our bad luck clung to us, but I was too busy with my report to assist much.

On 23 January 1899 Daniels forwarded a report on all this work to the "malaria investigation committee" of the Royal Society, which had sent him to me; and in this he confirmed every detail of my previous findings. By then, however, the matter had lost interest because my work had already been pirated by the Italians. For some reason best known to itself the Royal Society did not publish Daniels's report until 6 July 1900 (*Proceedings*). On 12 February he left me to join the other members of the Royal Society's malaria commission in Africa.

All this time plague had been gathering force in India and it still hampered us up to 1899. The authorities had fortunately been saved from the results of their previous want of preparation by possessing in Bombay the services of a man of genius, Mr W M W Haffkine, who had come to India to popularise his anticholera vaccine and had then invented his similar prophylactic against plague in 1896. But instead of giving him all the help he needed, they now appointed the usual commission "to examine and report." It consisted of Dr T R Fraser, an Edinburgh professor who had done good work on the cure of snake poison, Dr Almroth E Wright, professor of pathology at Netley, who had invented the important prophylactic against typhoid, and Dr M Armand Ruffer, a bacteriologist in Egypt. The two latter gentlemen visited Calcutta about Christmas 1898 and were, I think, sent to inspect my work "privately." We arranged to meet one morning in my laboratory but as I was a few minutes late they asked Daniels to show them the "pigmented cells." Unfortunately he was not yet fully acquainted with them and showed instead the nuclei of the cells of the mosquito's malpighian tubules. Ruffer detected the error at once and thought I was an impostor, and when I arrived there was almost a fracas! A specimen or two calmed it, however, and Wright and Ruffer ended by accepting my work fully—except the "black spores."

I have explained (page 185) what trouble those bodies caused me. Often I thought they were only parasites of parasites, but at other times, up to January 1899, I was almost convinced that they were really spores of the plasmodia, though I failed to get them to develop. Now Drs Wright and Ruffer supported the former hypothesis and Daniels the latter one; but before the end of the month I found numbers of the bodies in mosquitoes which had never been fed on infected blood at all and therefore expressed grave doubts as to their nature on the concluding page of my kala-azar report (30 January 1899). I was quite right to spend time over the question as it was not one to be summarily dismissed and has not been fully elucidated even yet. The subject of parasites of parasites is important apart from malaria. My work on kala-azar enlightened me on one point: the epidemiology of malaria could be fully explained on the supposition that the disease is communicated only from man to man by the mosquito—it was not necessary to assume further that mosquitoes infect each other and that they rise from the marsh already infected, as King had supposed (page 10). Hence the "black spores" were no longer necessary in the life cycle of the plasmodia.

Of course we showed Daniels all our technique and gave him all we knew about the habits of our mosquitoes—numerous facts, indeed, which I never published owing to my frequent interruptions. Of course all this was subsequently attributed to others who had really merely learnt from me; and Daniels consequently gave me the following letter upon the subject.

Letter from C W Daniels, MB, *Member of the Malaria Commission of the Royal Society and the Colonial Office*

8 *October* 1900.

Dear Ross,

I shall have great pleasure in testifying to the following facts:

1. Shortly after my arrival in Calcutta in December 1898 you showed me living specimens of your "grey," "brindled," and "dapple-winged" mosquitoes.

You pointed out to me the attitude assumed by the last, the position of its larva in water, and the peculiarities of its eggs.

Since then I have learnt that these are characteristics of the genus Anopheles.

You contrasted these with the eggs and larvae of other mosquitoes, which I now know to belong to the genus Culex.

2. You showed me two species of "dapple-winged" mosquitoes, and I sent specimens of them to the British Museum where they now are. They have been described by Major Giles, IMS, as anopheles.

You also showed me a specimen of the stomach of a mosquito with what are now known as "zygotes." This you stated was the stomach of a "dappled-winged" mosquito, similar to those you had shown me, which had been fed on a patient with crescents in 1897.

3. I may add that the development of proteosoma, as demonstrated to me by you in the "grey" mosquito, is essentially the same as the development of "crescents" in anopheles as observed by me in British Central Africa.

I am, yours very truly,
C W Daniels.

PS—As regards breeding places, you informed me that the "dapple-winged" mosquitoes breed in puddles, the "brindled" mosquitoes generally in flowerpots, and the "grey" mosquitoes in tanks, ditches, etc.

C W Daniels.

Major R Ross.

All these points are of fundamental importance in the theory of mosquito-borne diseases. About the same time the same facts were demonstrated by us to Dr F Plehn, a good German worker on malaria who spent several days at the laboratory. I do not think that I ever received a paper by him acknowledging this help, but certainly Daniels and he spread the cult widely from that time, since when everyone who ever saw a mosquito was able to rediscover the same facts for himself. To such the discovery of the facts is usually attributed in our learned textbooks on the subject. The plague scare was still so much in evidence that the colonel of a native regiment refused to allow Daniels, Plehn, and myself to examine his men.

During my year's special duty I received some, but not many, letters from people in India regarding my work. Among these were letters of congratulation from my old friends Surgeon Colonel Dobson and Surgeon Major John Smyth, then both at Bangalore. While I was still at Kherwara Dr Hayman Thornhill, senior medical officer of Ceylon, a real enthusiast on these subjects, offered to send me some living dapple-winged mosquitoes all the way from that island, but we decided that the idea was impracticable (at least, so far as I remember). Dr G Thin wrote me several pleasant letters in which he gradually dropped his mistaken estimate of the pigmented cells (page 132), though he never withdrew publicly his rather mischievous error. In the April number of the *Indian Medical Gazette* I had called attention to the need for a circulating medical library in Calcutta (fancy there being none!) and I have an interesting letter from that indefatigable and successful worker Captain (now Sir) Leonard Rogers, IMS, on the subject and another later one on kala-azar. I have several letters from Dr Maynard, who helped us by publishing our papers in the *Indian Medical Gazette*, of which he was editor, though I doubt whether he fully believed in Laveranity. I have three long ones from Surgeon Major G M Giles, IMS, who was then at home on furlough. He was courteous but entirely sceptical of the mosquito theory on rather feeble grounds, being evidently a good observer but a bad reasoner. My replies (copies of which I regret I do not possess) seem to have converted him, for some years later (1900) he produced his *Handbook of the Gnats, or Mosquitoes*,[44] which became the basis of malaria entomology. In this book he scarcely mentions my work except, very kindly, to apologise for my inaccuracies (2nd edition, page 153). When I met him some years later I asked him what precisely these inaccuracies were but found that he had never read my papers—or at least understood them! It was he who named *Anopheles rossi* after me because he "thought" they carried human malaria, though Daniels told him they did not. Nevertheless Giles was a valuable man and I wish I had had him with me in 1898. He never received a thankyou for his work. He mentioned my work as little as possible in his book and, *more Anglicano*, favoured the foreigners.

In June 1898 I had sent a copy of my proteosoma report[26] to Surgeon General Sternberg, the Director General of the Medical Department of the United States Army, and had written to him later giving my further results of July and August. I have no copy of my letter, but the reader may like to see the reply now in my possession, which proves that I had even then told the Americans how to reduce malaria by the methods which one of Sternberg's officers, W C Gorgas, employed so successfully some years later in Havana and Panama.

Subject: Causation of Fevers.

WAR DEPARTMENT, SURGEON GENERAL'S OFFICE,
WASHINGTON, *October* 14, 1898.

SURGEON MAJOR RONALD ROSS,
Indian Medical Service,
Care Postmaster, Calcutta, India.

SIR,

I am directed by the Surgeon General to acknowledge receipt of your interesting communication of August 24th last in relation to the causation of malarial fevers and to the practical deductions from your observations bearing on the suppression of such fevers by the use of mosquito nettings and satisfactory drainage.

No report has as yet been received from any of our medical officers on the causation of the fevers which affected our troops in Cuba and in the southern camps. Their energies so far have been wholly engaged in caring for the large number of sick men. Should any report be received bearing on your views the Surgeon General will have pleasure in sending you a copy.

Very respectfully,
(?) C STUART,
Deputy Surgeon General, USA

This letter was dated before a single person in the five continents had been able to repeat a single one of my observations on malaria and mosquitoes!

While I was in Nowgong permission at last reached me to publish my results (page 199). The letter was addressed to my chief from the Government of India, Home Department, 27 September 1898, and said that "the Government of India have no objection to Surgeon Major R Ross giving publicity to any results of his investigations connected with malarial fever after they have been duly communicated to you." Yet my chief had declared that the assent of the Secretary of State in London was required! All the trouble over my proteosoma report had therefore been, as my friends told me it was, quite unnecessary. But for Manson's expositions I might have lost priority for all my work on avian malaria. The letter mentioned above was really a snub for Leslie, who, I think, caused the trouble.

11

The Discovery Discovered. Calcutta, 1898–1899

THE lay reader who is not acquainted with the niceties of scientific priority may be surprised that I should insist so freqently on mine. He will know the reason soon because I have now to describe the discovery of my work in Europe—*indipendentemente da Ross*.

As stated on page 164, my proteosoma report[26] had been sent out in June 1898 to a number of people—Manson, Laveran, Metchnikoff, Thin, Giles, Sternberg, the president of the Royal Society, the medical press, and elsewhere—about 30 or 40 copies. This report described the necessary technique and figured the pigmented cells completely up to, but not including, sporulation. The rest of the life cycle was described in detail by Manson before a large audience of the British Medical Association at the end of July,[46] all the facts being given in the *Lancet* of 20 August, while Manson's full paper, with a number of illustrations, including some of the germinal threads in the salivary glands of mosquitoes, appeared in the *British Medical Journal* of 24 September 1898, of which many thousands of copies were issued. Besides all this, I had sent scores of my specimens and mosquitoes to Manson and to Laveran, and on 7 October the latter had written to me from the Pasteur Institute of Paris—the recognised world centre for such studies:

"*Je vous remercie sincèrement de votre très intéressante lettre du 2 Sept. qui confirme et complète, sur plusieurs points importants, vos précédentes lettres.... Les résultats des infections expérimentals, obtenus chez des oiseaux sains, sont très remarquables; je vous félicite d'avoir résolu ce difficile problème.*" After this there would be no trouble whatever in repeating the same work for any of the parasites, human or avian; and how anyone could have the impudence to pretend to do so independently of me would be a mystery outside pure charlatanism.

How easily the work could be repeated, given time and opportunity, was proved in August 1899 when, within a few days of landing in Sierra Leone, I was able to demonstrate the development of all three species of human plasmodia in two kinds of "dapple-wings," *Anopheles costalis* and *A funestus*. On 6 September 1898 (as already quoted) I had told Manson that it would be easy to infect healthy men experimentally by the bites of mosquitoes by my method, and on 31 October I wrote:

"You must not trouble yourself in the least about obtaining confirmation of my mosquito work. Before another year has passed there will be dozens of workers all over the world. There is really no difficulty at all *except finding the right hosts* for each species of parasite. A few years more and the whole business will be established as the most beautiful of all the processes of nature in connection with disease. Malaria from beginning to end will be the 'show' disease."

All this happened. My storm-tost treasure-bark had now safely crossed the wide solitary ocean and was approaching harbour; but it was soon to be surrounded by a clamour of pilot boats and steam tugs all offering to navigate me in (on payment), and the pirates lay in the offing ready to board me at the proper moment!

The current facts were supplied to me in two series of amusing letters from Dr G H F Nuttall and Dr Edmonston Charles. The first man to venture forth was the great Robert Koch, of Berlin, the discoverer of the cause of tuberculosis and of cholera, who first established bacteriology as a practical science by his plate culture methods. On 2 September 1898 Manson wrote to me:

"Koch has gone to Rome to study malaria. Pity he didn't go there before. I sent him one of your reports which the India Office sent me.... I also learn officially that Koch and a commission are going out to India [and] Africa [illegible] for two years to study malaria.... Doubtless your mosquito discoveries have instigated this move. In his later lucubrations Koch claims the mosquito as his own and never says a word about your work. Cool is it not?"

On 6 October Manson wrote to me:

"A great many of your slides have perished utterly, some are deteriorating rapidly. A good many are still in good preservation, but I fear for their future. I am sending one to Rome in a day or two. I hear that Bignami and Marchiafava are going into the country to work mosquitoes and I also hear that the American pack is in full cry after the mosquito."

On 30 October he wrote: "I hear Koch has failed with the mosquito in Italy so you have time to grab the discovery for England"—he meant to complete human malaria in the mosquito. Similarly Laveran, in his letter of 12 September, told me that Koch admitted malaria infection by mosquitoes but that he had not added more evidence in favour of this. I did not know of Dr Nuttall until I received his first letter. He said:

ALTONAIRSTRASSE, BERLIN, N W,
13 *August* 1898.

DEAR SIR,

... Whilst in London lately I called on Dr Manson, who was very kind, and we spent an evening over your preparations, one of which he has since kindly sent me. I have just written a review of your remarkable researches for one of the German journals, the *Hygienische Rundschau*, feeling that people here ought to know more about them. Dr Manson sent me your "Report on the Cultivation of Proteosoma Labbé in Grey Mosquitoes," and in a letter has told me of your last beautiful observation of the parasite in the salivary glands of the mosquito.... I am at present engaged in a lengthy paper in which I give a critical and historical review of our present knowledge of the part played by insects in infectious diseases.... I shall be publishing it in English as well as in German and shall have the pleasure of sending you a copy in due time. The mosquito-malarial theory (?) will be discussed at length and your work too. Koch, who came back recently from German East Africa, declares himself in favour of the theory and says it would be very important to follow up the matter experimentally on mosquitoes. He ignores your work completely. I have just written a review of his publication and have drawn attention to this.... Hoping that you will reap the reward of your brilliant and painstaking researches in the shape of suitable encouragement from the goverment, I remain, my dear Dr Ross.

Yours very sincerely,
GEO H F NUTTALL.

He also made me some suggestions which I had already considered. I did not like to hear all this of Koch, who was to me a star of the first magnitude, and I could not conceive how he or any man of fame could plagiarise the work of an obscure person like myself; but it was evident that scientific morality was not as impeccable as I thought. When, however, Koch's article[53] appeared in 1899 he gave me full credit in a single sentence, though he did not mention Manson's theory.* He confirmed all my proteosoma work and described the movements of the "vermiculi," which I had no time to examine; but he did not deal with the human plasmodia. He had thought of the mosquito theory as early as 1883–4 and now cultivated proteosoma in Rome in September 1898—see his letter to me on page 73 of my Nobel Lecture.[17]

Nuttall's subsequent letters to me gave chiefly several criticisms of my nomenclature and some suggestions, one or two of which would have been useful if I could have continued my work. I explained that my terms such as "proteosoma coccidia" and "germinal threads" were, like "grey mosquito" and "dapple-winged mosquito," merely provisional, as I could obtain no scientific advice on the subject in India.

Now for the Italian work. As already quoted, Manson told me on 6 October that he was sending one of my specimens to Rome. He sent two to Dr T Edmonston Charles, a retired Deputy Surgeon General (? IMS), who was living there. After this Drs A Bignami and C Bastianelli and Professor B Grassi of that city gradually carried out for Italy the local researches which I had always considered would constitute the necessary second part of my investigation—that was, to extend my general results to local parasites and mosquitoes; but they were able to do so only in the light of my work and not, as they pretended, independently of me. Seven months later I did the same for Sierra Leone—and would have done so had Koch, Bignami, Bastianelli, and Grassi never existed. The reader who is jealous for the honour and welfare of science, as I am, should follow the facts. I will give here only some of them as they became known to me. The piracy has now become merely ludicrous, but nevertheless it is my duty to expose it once more in this book.

* His exact words were:
"Die Erforschung der Malariaätiologie hat drei wichtige Entdeckungen aufzuweisen:
"1. Die Entdeckung der Malariaparasiten durch Laveran;
"2. Die Entdeckung des Entwickelungsganges der Malariaparasiten innerhalb des eigentlichen Wirthes, d.h. im Körper des erkrankten Menschen durch Golgi und
"3. Die Entdeckung der Entwickelung der Malariaparasiten ausserhalb des menschlichen, bezw. thierischen Körpers im Zwischenwirth, in der Stechmücke durch Ross."

21, QUEEN ANNE STREET, CAVENDISH SQUARE, W.,
8 *November*, 1898.

MY DEAR ROSS,

Charles writes me he has given you the great news from the Imperial City. You are now on the mounting wave which I trust will surely lead on to fortune. Bignami should have experimented on your lines though. He ought to have fed his mosquitoes on crescent blood, waited a week for the germinal bodies to form, and then set them to bite. I have written Charles to tell him this and I hope he will not be too late this season to try. I hope, however, you have anticipated him and that you can give chapter and verse—that is, mosquito and experiment for tertian, quartan, and crescent malaria—by this time....

I sent Bignami and Charles one of your preparations each. I grudge to part with them, but I think it is in your interest that the Romans should have ocular proof that you have been before them. I fear that these furrineers [*sic*] are inclined to filch as much as they can. This is a sentiment I only breathe to you. We will take care that your interests are looked after here....

I hope you are feeling better and that you are able to place the top stone on your magnificent building.

Yours sincerely,
PATRICK MANSON.

Dr Charles's letters were all typewritten.

72 VIA DI SAN NICCOLO DA TOLENTINO, ROME,
November 4, 1898.

DEAR DR ROSS,

Dr Crombie stayed with me at Upper Norwood this summer and I went north to Glen Urquhart to stay with him. Naturally we discussed your work much and Crombie was to have given me an introduction to you, but the second visit he intended to pay me did not come off and I had to leave London without any letter for you, and for the moment I do not know Dr Crombie's address.

I called on Dr Manson before leaving London to get the latest news of what progress you had made in your work in order to let the Italians know. They have been working in various directions this summer, but up till this week without being able to show any definite results. Bignami has collected mosquitoes from four very malarious localities.

According to Grassi it would seem there are some 50 varieties of mosquito in Italy. Only six, however, seem to frequent these selected malarial positions.

Besides the mosquitoes, the larvae were also brought up and allowed to develop in Rome.

Four different persons were shut up again and again in a room with a number of these mosquitoes. The experiments extended over months till at last a success has just been met with.*

Besides these experiments, Bignami has been studying the question of the flagella with great care. As he has found chromatin in some but not all of the flagella† distributed irregularly, he will soon have to make up his mind to abandon the position he took up, that only degenerated forms of the plasmodium gave rise to flagellation.

Celli has been working at the subject of rendering men immune to malaria. He has been using the serum of immune animals and extract of the internal organs. His results have not been published, but there is an idea abroad that he has met with partial success.

Koch is not in Rome now, but though I tried hard to find out what he had been doing I can get hardly any information. He seems to have been very silent as to his work and to have refused to speak about it. It may interest you, however, to know that he spoke in the highest terms regarding your work and also that he looks upon the flagellum as being some kind of spore.

My friend Dr Brock looks upon the movement that he sees in the pigment of the body before flagellation takes place as indicating the flagella are moving about before they become extruded.

By the same post I send you a copy of a lay paper, the *Tribuna*, bearing today's date. In the article I have marked it is stated that Grassi holds that only three species of mosquito are capable of conveying malarial fever. It is also stated that one of Bignami's patients developed fever two days after having been bitten by these mosquitoes and that yesterday, for the first time, malarial parasites were found in his blood. Immediately after this the patient took quinine.

From my conversation a week ago with Bignami I satisfied myself that if he got any successes we could rely on his careful experiments as excluding error. I for one, therefore, accept his position without hesitation. I have been three times today to try and catch him at his laboratory but was unsuccessful in finding him. I will go again, however,

* But only after change of procedure (page 213).

† This had already been done by N Sakharoff.[31]

before the post leaves in case any other patient that he has been experimenting with may have developed fever.

In the *Tribuna* it is mentioned that Dionisi has found in bats malarial infection caused by parasites similar to those of human malaria. This observation of his has still to be followed out.

Although I have sent you the *Tribuna*, unless it is easy for you to have it translated do not do so. I have picked out all the points that will interest you.

I have told Professor Marchiafava that I will write and ask you for specimens of the mosquito in which human malaria develops.* Also for those which you use with regard to bird malaria. They will send them to Grassi to be identified with the Italian mosquito. I suggested to Bignami that they might be sent in formalin. He said, however, that it was better to dry them and make mummies of them. He seems to think that the formalin injures the ornaments and other finer structures. Perhaps, however, it will be safer to send them in both ways.

We would also prize much any of your bird malaria or other preparations. If the Italians can only see your results it may stir them up to follow in your footsteps.

Naturally you would like to have your work confirmed by men who have done such good pioneering already. Of course you must guard yourself against sending us any specimens regarding which you have not published your results.

It has been a cause of surprise to me how very closely they have followed all that you have done and how fluently they talk regarding details of your work.† I need not assure you with what pride all Englishmen follow all you do. In Edinburgh Manson's quiet exposition of your latest results created quite a furore.

Though ill and suffering, he unfolded the story with great completeness and effect.

Yours very truly,
T Edmonston Charles.

PS—I did not find Bignami at his laboratory and called at his house after dark with no better success. If I can get any details out of him likely to interest you I shall send them to you by next mail.

I received both these letters shortly after my return to Calcutta.

* Yet Grassi denied later that I had ever found this mosquito.

† Yet Grassi stated later that his labours were independent of mine.

Bignami had evidently infected a man just as I told Manson in my letter of 6 September Koch was likely to do. The announcement was received by me with mixed feelings: I had long wished to crown my work by infecting myself with an infected mosquito (quinine was always at hand to cure me), but on the other hand was now saved this disagreeable triumph and was glad to obtain such corroboration of my labours. With Dr Edmonston Charles I was not acquainted, but as I knew the poor reputation of these Italian gentlemen in connection with the work of Laveran and Golgi I confess that at first I thought him to be a busybody who was trying to get unpublished information from me for the advantage of questionable friends and I was correspondingly reserved in my reply.

It will be remembered (page 75) that in 1896 Bignami had opposed Manson's induction but had at the same time tried to substitute another theory, that mosquitoes bring the plasmodia from marshes and inject them into men by their bite[30]; and he added that some years previously he had tried to verify this theory by causing mosquitoes brought from a malarious locality (? larvae or adults) to bite healthy men but had failed. Since then we had heard no more of Italian work on the mosquito theory; but now that our papers of 18 December 1897, 26 February, and 18 June 1898 and Manson's address at Edinburgh on 28 July 1898 were known to all we expected further developments. Bignami says[33] that he began to resume his experiments (doubtless *indipendentemente da Ross*) early in August following—that is, *possibly* before he had heard of Manson's announcement of the infection of birds by me. Anyway he proceeded chiefly by bringing *larvae* from stagnant pools in the Campagna, hatching them out in Rome, and causing the *adults* to bite two men, G N and A S, for many nights. Both cases remained quite negative of course, and he would probably have continued similar futile experiments indefinitely but for Manson's address on my work,[46] which showed that infecting mosquitoes must be themselves infected by biting birds or men after being hatched from the larva—published in the *Lancet* of 30 August and the *British Medical Journal* of 24 September. His third experiment, therefore (which he says was commenced on 26 September) was done with *adult* mosquitoes, including *Culex penicillaris*, Grassi's "*Culex malariae*," and *Anopheles claviger* (*maculipennis*), collected from Maccarese, a malarious place in the Campagna (he does not say how). The patient, A S (Sola), began to have fever on 31 October and *Plasmodium falciparum* was said to be found in him on 3 November. He had probably been infected by the *A claviger*, which had previously bitten infected persons at Maccarese. The experiment was thus really only a repetition of my experiments on birds carried out three months previously. It was of little scientific value, but Bignami claimed to have entirely proved the mosquito theory by it!

His paper[33] appeared on 15 November and a translation of it called "The inoculation theory of malarial infection: account of a successful experiment with mosquitoes" was published in the *Lancet* of 3 and 10 December 1898—reaching me about the end of the year. It was a wordy, confused paper, cleverly written so as to conceal the author's obligation to us. In order to avoid this charge of concealment he mentions and praises my work up to Manson's announcement[46] of July 1898; but also, in order to avoid the obligation, he gives no clear account of my work nor even of my infection of healthy birds, nor does he explain the real reason why he changed his experimental procedure (from the use of mosquito larvae to that of adults) in September for his third experiment—a vital and fundamental change. He leaves it to be inferred by the ignorant reader that his success was independent of my work and due to the same kind of experiment as those which he had used in 1894—which was not the case. And of course he completely ignores the zoological rule of priority, that the life cycle of *Plasmodium relicta* proteosoma covers that of *P falciparum*. Personally I would not care to write such a paper.

The Roman writers possessed many advantages over me. They were free to do as they pleased; they could publish their results a few days after obtaining them; there were numerous well known intensely malarious spots close at hand; and there were many hospitals and laboratories and professors to consult if necessary. Above all, their mosquitoes were already classified and described in Ficalbi's monograph of the Italian Culicidae[21] while I could obtain no information whatever on the subject in India. Lastly they had good libraries and all my experience and writing to guide them. To continue Charles's letters then:

72 Via di San Niccolo da Tolentino, Rome,
November 19, 1898.

Dear Dr Ross,

Since my letter dated the 4th they have had no more successes in conveying infection through the mosquito.

The fact is, the Vienna plague outbreak has made it very difficult to persuade people to allow themselves to be bitten by mosquitoes.

As, doubtless, it would help you to have named specimens of the mosquitoes spoken of by Grassi, I went to his laboratory to try and get him to give you a few specimens of the different kinds of mosquito.

I did this under the impression that he had completed his investigations. He told me, however, they were far from complete and did not give me the specimens.

He spoke in the highest terms of praise of your work; he has your first report* and told me to write to try and get your future reports at an early date for him. I therefore write to India for them today.

Late last night Grassi sent me a note on malaria propagated by special insects. He presented it to the Royal Academy of the Lincei on the 6th of November.† It had not been published the day before yesterday. As the post goes this forenoon I have just run my eye over it and send you the following extracts:

He thinks the grey mosquitoes you sent him are *Culex pipiens*. The word mosquito is a vulgar term that includes many diverse and, in part, many different genera of insects (Culex, Anopheles, Aedes, Ceratopogon, Simulia, Phlebotomus). The included species amount to many over a hundred.

Briefly, his previous researches may be arranged in a résumé thus: (1) The Ceratopogon, the Simulia, the Aedes, and the Phlebotomos are, at the least, not necessary for malarial infection. (2) Certain species of mosquito, amongst which the most common, *Culex pipiens*, ought to be held innocuous. (3) Certain other species are at the least not necessary—*Culex richiardii*, *Culex annulatus*, *Culex hortensis*, *Anopheles bifurcatus*, *Anopheles nigripes*, *Culex spathipalpis*, *Culex pulchritarsis*. (4) Certain species are under great suspicion; these are the following—*Anopheles claviger Fabr*, *Culex penicillaris*, *Culex malariae*. My servant,‡ who was infected with malaria, was only bitten by these three species in the month preceding infection. I was thus led to the conclusion that the first two, at least the second, possibly even the third, ordinarily furnished the alternating host of the malarial parasite of man.

Bignami's first ineffectual experiments seemed to have been conducted with *Culex pipiens* and perhaps with *Culex hortensis*.

It may be asked, are all the three species to blame, or two, or only one

* On the cultivation of proteosoma,[26] containing full details of my technique etc; sent by Manson.

† See References[54].

‡ Charles is here evidently quoting direct from Grassi, though there are no quotation marks in his letter.

of them? I suspect, and also say that I believe it to be ascertained, that *Culex penicillaris* propagates malarial fever. I cannot, however, in fact deny that the other two forms do the same.

In order to infect, malarial mosquitoes must themselves be infected. The greater number of them are certainly not so.

All that we know of the cycles of evolution of animal parasites makes us affirm that marsh moquitoes are the only way of the transmission of malaria.*

In a polemic on the subject Grassi published a letter in the *Corriere della Sera* of the 13th November in which he boldly states that it is quite unnecessary to have resort to the hypothesis of malarial germs in the soil.

Grassi showed me in the blood of the owl two small parasites, very slightly pigmented, which I could not distinguish from the summer-autumn parasite of human malaria. This, together with Dionisi's observation of quartan and summer-autumn parasites in bats, opens out a huge vista for careful investigation. One difficulty of accepting without reserve the mosquito theory was the fact that malaria seems to abound where there are no men. If bats, owls, and possibly other twilight feeders furnish the appropriate intermediate hosts for malarial parasites man may be considered as a mere accidental host. Man suffers when the spores with their attendant toxins are discharged from the red blood corpuscle. Sporulation does not seem to have been noticed in bats or owls, hence they do not seem to suffer much from affording a resting place for the parasite.

It would be very interesting if you could go a little into this inquiry. Probably, if man is an accidental host and the night-feeding mammal or bird the really natural host of the parasite, it would seem to be extremely likely that you get the parasite to develop in the mosquito more easily from one of the night-feeding creatures than from man. Anyhow, if you have the same difficulty in getting subjects to allow themselves to be bitten by artificially infected mosquitoes bats, owls, etc will prove a godsend to you.

I have been trying for some days to get the bookseller to procure for

* Quotation apparently ends. All these opinions on the species of mosquito concerned in malaria were mere guesses without scientific evidence and were mostly wrong. Yet Grassi subsequently claimed to have found the "*Anopheles malariferi*" independently of me, not only for Italy but for the whole world, *solely* on the strength of these bogus conjectures; and a number of incompetent writers still credit him with the achievement!

me a copy of Ficalbi on the various species of the European culex. He has not yet found it for me. If I can get a copy I will try and translate for you the description he gives of some of the species referred to by Grassi.

Grassi seems very friendly, and several times he assured me that if you sent him any specimens of mosquitoes he would name and classify them for you.

It seems there are many grey mosquitoes besides *Culex pipiens*. One dappled-winged mosquito is *Anopheles claviger*.*

Grassi would like dried specimens sent in a pillbox with a little naphthalene. He particularly wants males as well as females. These resemble the female but have ornaments on the proboscis which prevent them from biting.

Grassi would also like some specimens sent in alcohol. If Grassi can name us a certain number of mosquitoes for you it will enable you to follow future Italian work with more exactness as they will doubtless all name the mosquito with which they are working.

Yours very truly,
T Edmonston Charles.

72 Via di San Niccolo da Tolentino, Rome,
November 25, 1898.

Dear Mr Ross,

I went to Professor Grassi's laboratory and showed him one of your preparations (third day, from the sparrow) showing pigments etc in the walls of the mosquito's stomach. He seemed much pleased and I understood him to say he had just found it in a preparation of his own† and that in a week he hoped to have verified all you work.

He had before him the *British Medical Journal* with your paper of the 18th December 1897 and seemed perfectly satisfied that your description of the mosquito referred to *Anopheles claviger*.‡ He had numbers of these

* They had recognised the genus by the eggs *plus* the wing-marks.

† This statement of Grassi's does not agree withthe opening sentence of Charles's next letter. What a pity that the former did not show his specimen to the latter at the same time!

‡ Which carries malaria in Italy. Yet afterwards Grassi said that he found it independently of me. *A claviger* has nearly the same eggs and wing marks as my large dapple-wing, in which I first cultivated human malaria 15 months previously (page 113). Evidently Charles also was familiar with my paper.[42]

mosquitoes in a bottle and volunteered to give me one to send to you. He had no males, but I send you two females by today's post. This mosquito, however, seems darker in colour than the one you describe; although you use the word "dark brown" species to designate it, I note that lower down you say that the back of the thorax and the abdomen is a light fawn colour.

In a previous letter I told you that at the Santo Spirito they looked upon *Anopheles claviger* as your dapple-wing, which, of course, it is not.* On my mentioning to Grassi that they had not succeeded at the S Spirito at finding any development in *Anopheles claviger* after feeding it both on spring tertian blood and on blood containing summer-autumn parasite (the blood was apparently favourable as I found crescents in the one fever case and large flagella-producing forms in the spring tertian) Grassi threw out the suggestion that, as the mosquitoes had bitten in a cold ward, the sudden change from the warm blood of the man to the cold stomach of the mosquito may have been too much for the parasite and inhibited the changes wished for. Grassi breeds his mosquitoes in a small room with a stove; the temperature felt to me over 80 ° F. At the time of the experiment in the S Spirito I should judge the temperature to be just over 60 ° F, having as a guide the temperature in my own house at that time. In your future reports it would help to throw light on this point if you stated the temperature at which you worked. If in very cold weather you can procure a case of malaria you might heat up a small room by lamps or otherwise to put your fever patient in during one of your experiments.

Bignami has written a paper, not yet published, which Dr Brock is translating for the *Lancet*. I have asked him to try and get me some reprints of it as it is so much more handy for reference in this form. If he succeeds they ought to be here in about a fortnight and I will send you a copy.

Bignami's one success in producing fever through the bites of mosquitoes will be described in it and a good many speculations and clever arguments are sure to be gathered together. Besides this, the finding of chromatin in the flagella and the probable import of this discovery will be dwelt on.

Yours very truly,

T Edmonston Charles.

PS I send you a translation of Grassi's first paper.

* Not the same species but the same genus.

72 Via di San Niccolo da Tolentino, Rome,
December 2, 1898.

Dear Dr Ross,

Within four or five hours of posting your letter last week they found your pigmented bodies in the walls of the stomach of a mosquito.* It had been fed on crescents.

On the 28th November their success was reported to the Royal Academy of the Lincei, as appears from a reprint which I send you by today's book post from the authors. I send you also a translation of this communication. You will see they report success up to the fourth day. Since then they have only advanced to the sixth day and consequently have not met with your germinal rods.

For some days they have had a great mortality amongst their mosquitoes but they tell me today that they have succeeded better in keeping them alive. I fancy this must be due to their following your tactics more closely as regards feeding, water, and daily change of tubes.†

Bignami gave me a copy of his new paper yesterday; there are 31 pages of it. I have just had time to run my eye over it. There is nothing of much importance that you should know at once. In fact I have referred to almost every point in my previous letters. He defines very clearly his position with regard to the flagella and seems ready, as soon as proof can be secured by experiment, to throw over both air and water as media of communication of malaria.

If you have plenty of material you would help much in settling the question by making people breathe dry germinal rods and others drink them. This question is so important and, in a sense, constitutes a part of your inquiry that I do not hesitate to urge it on you.‡

The season is too far advanced and the material too scanty for the Italians to achieve much more success. I have told them how pleased you will be to hear that such competent specialists have been able to confirm your work. Perhaps with their report in your hand it might suit you to mention the fact in your next communication to the government.

I fear we shall not be able to get your third report till well on in February, and that is a long time to wait.

If you can spare 10 minutes do tell us in half a dozen lines what

* *A claviger*, which they thought was my "dapple-wing"!

† These clever gentlemen never mention such trifles in their papers.

‡ Like advising a cobbler to make boots.

progress you have made, especially whether you have been able to trace the germinal rods in man's malaria and whether you have succeeded in producing fever through bites of artificially infected mosquitoes.

You know already that they have failed in cultivating quartan fever in *Anopheles claviger*. Apparently their previous failure with crescents may have depended upon the crescents being immature, as they had only just begun to form in the case experimented with.

If you chance to be anywhere with quartans and tertians abounding I fancy you will not have much difficulty in recognising what mosquito you ought to work with as the species causing the mischief should also be abundant.

I do not know whether I should allude to the fact that, in their communication of the 28th November, a suspicion of doubt is hinted at as to whether, possibly, your two mosquitoes before they fed on man had not previously bitten some other animal.* From a purely scientific point of view I suppose it is impossible to disprove this suggestion; at any rate it can display no animus against you as all three writers acknowledge unreservedly the vast importance of your work and the great successes that you have achieved. Grassi, in fact, every time he sees me, again and again is jubilant in his praises.† He does not seem to be making any progress in confirming what you have published about the proteosoma. He cannot get *Culex pipiens* to bite and thinks that they are too young as yet.

Under mosquito nets they have large numbers of *Anopheles claviger*. They seem to be more successful in keeping them alive in this state of comparative freedom than imprisoned in test tubes so there seems to be a possibility of procuring enough material to continue their studies for some time longer.

I shall send you some more translation if ready in time for today's mail, otherwise by next week's mail.

Yours very truly,
T Edmonston Charles.

The success reported at the beginning of this last letter was obtained with *Anopheles claviger* Fabr, also called *A maculipennis* Meig and *A quadrimaculatus*, Say the common Anopheles of Europe and other

* Yet Charles and his friends must have seen the second sentence in my paper which they had all read and *studied carefully* and in which I stated that my mosquitoes were "bred in bottles from the larva" (see page 222).

† Yet his researches were independent of mine.

countries. The Italians had already recognised my "dapple-winged mosquitoes" to belong to this genus from the description of the *four spots* on the wings and the peculiar boat-shaped eggs given in my paper of 18 December 1897, in which I first described finding the pigmented cells in a species of this group (page 233). The Italian success was therefore merely a confirmation of my original discovery of the human plasmodia in anopheles made on 20 August 1897, 15 months previously. Any honest men of science would, of course, have said so in the very beginning of their paper, but Messrs Bastianelli, Bignami, and Grassi reported the matter a few days later[55] as follows (in Dr Charles's translation):

Royal Academy of the Lincei

Medical Zoology.—Cultivation of the malarial crescents of man in *Anopheles claviger* Fabr. (Synonym *Anopheles maculipennis* Meig). (Submitted 28 November 1898.) Preliminary note by G Bastianelli, A Bignami, and B Grassi, presented by the associate B Grassi.

We have proposed to study the relationship between the special species of mosquito and the special species of parasite in the malaria of man, and having regard to the complexity of the undertaking we have judged it opportune to work together. As the first result of our researches we can announce that we have been able to follow with all certainty certain phases of the development of the semilunar bodies in the thickness of the middle intestine of several (other*) *Anopheles claviger*, kept at a favourable temperature, which we have made to suck the blood of individuals affected with the summer-autumnal form of malaria.

The most notable phases in question find a comparison in those discovered by Ross (second and third day) for the proteosoma (haemamoeba) of birds.

In a room containing four malarial patients (all affected with aestivo-autumnal fever?) we have collected: six *Culex pipiens*, one *Anopheles nigripes*, four *Anopheles claviger*.

The examination of these Culicidae led to a negative result except in the cases of two of the *Anopheles claviger*, in which we found the further stages of development corresponding to those described by Ross for the proteosoma of birds (fourth day). Apparently the two mosquitoes with *spotted* wings (note: there exist in Europe five species of culex with spotted wings. In India we do not know of any data) in which Ross

* Not in the original. R R.

found in India the stages of development similar to those of the proteosoma (about the third day) belonged also to the species *Anopheles claviger* Fabr.

Ross, however, not having followed the development of these bodies, could not with certainty refer them to the crescents, it being also possible that his two mosquitoes, before having bitten men, had already bitten another animal.

Up till now many other attempts to cultivate the parasites of owls and pigeons have given negative results in *Anopheles claviger*.

We have to note in conclusion that at Lentini (Sicily) during the months of October and November malaria prevailed much, but *Culex penicillaris* and *Culex malariae* were not to be found; *Anopheles claviger* on the other hand was extraordinarily abundant.

It will be observed:

1. That these people do not mention where exactly my work was published so that their hearers or readers could not verify their statements regarding it.

2. Their statement that "it [is] also possible that his two mosquitoes, before having bitten men, had already bitten another animal" was directly contrary to the second sentence in my paper in the *British Medical Journal*,[42] 18 December 1897, in which I said: "For the last two years I have been endeavouring to cultivate the parasite of malaria in the mosquito. The method adopted has been to feed mosquitoes, *bred in bottles from the larva*, on patients having crescents in the blood and then to examine their tissues for parasites similar to the haemamoeba in man." The rest of my paper reported the finding of such parasites; and the whole case was fully proved by my subsequent work on human and avian parasites.

3. Messrs Bastianelli, Bignami, and Grassi must have had this paper of mine before them when they wrote their note (see Charles, page 217). Their statement was therefore a deliberate and intentional lie told in order to discredit my work and so to obtain the priority for themselves and constantly reiterated even after I had exposed it.

4. It is amusing to observe that they themselves say nothing about their own mosquitoes having been bred from the larva. Also they had succeeded only with two insects! Yet they demand "all certainty" for their observations, which they refuse for mine.

5. The falsification is so obvious that one may doubt the truth of the whole *nota preliminare* given above. It is quite *possible* that these gentlemen were at that time merely showing my preparations which Manson had sent them.

Their next paper[56] was dated 22 December 1898 and was published by the same academy. It describes the finding of "pigmented cells" in some more *Anopheles claviger* but does not state exactly in how many or whether the insects used had been bred from the larvae. In fact the article might have been transcribed bodily from my proteosoma report and Manson's Edinburgh address. My name is mentioned only once, on the fifth page, where the three authors say (again in Charles's translation): "The observations reported up till now permit us to reconstruct the life cycle of the human haemosporidia in the body of *Anopheles claviger*: it finds for the most part confirmation in that observed by Ross regarding the proteosoma of birds in the *grey mosquito*." In other words, my work confirmed that of these rascals! Again, no exact references to my writings are given.

From the intrinsic evidence of these two papers I believe with Koch that it is quite *possible* that the alleged observations were never really made at all but that the papers were written entirely from my specimens and descriptions in order to obtain priority for the discovery of the human parasites in anophelines—which the writers then thought I was making in India. More *probably*, however, they did find the pigmented cells but only in some old *Anopheles claviger* which had been *caught in rooms* where malaria cases were sleeping—as, in fact, they actually say in their second *nota preliminare*—that is, just as I found the cells some months later in *Anopheles costalis* caught in Wilberforce Barracks in Sierra Leone. Some of these old *A claviger* may have been refed subsequently on the malaria cases in hospital; but in neither *nota preliminare* is there any statement whatever that the insects employed had been bred from the larvae in captivity and then fed on the malaria cases in hospital for the first time—no such statement, in fact, as I had clearly made in my article of 18 December 1897. Thus the very ambiguity which the authors falsely asserted against my work existed in their own papers when they made the assertion. Of course the plasmodial nature of the pigmented cells in their mosquitoes was guaranteed "with all certainty" not by any work of theirs but by my preceding proofs of the whole life cycle of proteosoma in mosquitoes. Can any more impudent scientific frauds than these two preliminary notes of Messrs Grassi, Bignami, and Bastianelli be imagined?

This sort of thing is not uncommon in science, which it impedes and disgraces. All cases of it ought to be publicly exposed when detected and I therefore do not mince my words regarding the present one.

Dr Charles wrote me four more letters from Rome up to 14 January 1899—they need not be given here. When I received his three first letters

I did not appreciate exactly what had happened and consequently wrote him a very gentle corrective reply on 19 December. But when I received the fourth one (of 2 December) the piracy became manifest and I criticised the Italian work somewhat shortly and closed the correspondence. Similarly I thought well of Grassi at first and in my paper for the *Institut Pasteur* (which was finished on 31 December 1898) actually said that he was working independently of us! I had not seen all his papers then, and indeed he did not fully develop his ingenious strategy till he wrote his book, published in June 1900. I soon heard, however, that the brigands had fallen out over their booty; but I now leave them in full enjoyment of it.

On 13 December I sent Charles some specimens of proteosoma, some grey mosquitoes, and a dapple-winged one. On 19 November he wrote two surprising offical letters, to the India Office and to the Government of India respectively, asking for immediate copies of my reports and for specimens from me and saying how familiar the Italians were with my work and so on. These letters reached me (as official prints) in February 1899 and I was commanded to do as Dr Charles wished. My friends blamed Charles for writing them—I am sure that he acted in good faith but was used as a cat's-paw by his clever acquaintances.

Hitherto I had always passionately denied the truth of Tennyson's lines:

> The man of science himself is fonder of glory, and vain,
> An eye well-practised in nature, a spirit bounded and poor.

But now I felt like one who has long been living with distinguished and agreeable friends whom he suddenly finds to be a gang of sordid adventurers. Science was never the same again to me.

Of course Manson knew all about these doings. On 7 December he wrote: "You will see from the *Lancet* the position Bignami is taking and how there is an attempt to belittle you while exalting himself. All this is very amusing and contemptible.... You have plenty of friends here who know how to uphold you and your rights. Your work is the starting point of all this mosquito business." On 10 January he wrote very kindly: "You have forged the key and others must take the trouble to open the door ... we will take care here that your position in this matter is not ignored.... That kala-azar business was most unfortunate. Had you been left alone you would have anticipated all that the Italians are doing. Practically you had already done it and you can justly claim to have been the first to find the malaria parasite in the mosquito as well as to point out the *modus operandi* of that insect in diffusing malaria.... Two mails ago I wrote to Harvey telling him that I hoped he would get the Indian Government to make some recognition of the splendid work you have done. I pointed out that its enormous importance was already recognised in Europe and that honours were in store for you here. I told him that it would be a graceful act for the Indian Government to anticipate these. I also wrote in the same strain to Colonel Fenn, whom I know, to influence the Viceroy in the same direction." On 18 January he wrote: "The Romans are still active. I wrote last week to Bignami telling him we were careful of your reputation and hoping that he and his compatriots would be equally so. They are all on the grab it would seem. I had a letter from Charles today saying that there are now some 20 or thereby claimants for the mosquito theory. I dare say in another month there will be 50.... But don't let your wish for completeness keep you a day longer in India than your health will stand. Don't risk anything. Your work is practically complete and you should come home for a time.... They are getting up a tropical school in Liverpool and came to me about a lecturer etc. Amongst others I suggested your name and Boyce has jumped at the idea."

These were the last letters that Manson wrote to me in India— noble series such as few men had received.

I do not think that when he wrote to Bignami (of course, without effect) he could have read with attention the later Italian papers. My complaint was not that the Italians had anticipated me regarding the completion of the human malaria work—a trifling matter—but that they had sullied science by misrepresenting the facts. In spite of Manson's statements above I can remember little exposure of this in the scientific press at home. I still possess the draft of a letter to the *British Medical Journal* in which I mildly attempted to expose the Italian doings. It was sent in before 5 January 1899 (my letter to Manson of that date) but for some reason was never published. No English periodical ever published my remonstrances and none of my English friends ever fought for me. I was obliged at last to carry the fight into Italy. The *Indian Medical Gazette* of March 1899, however, protested strongly against the piracy. I do not know for certain who wrote the article but am much indebted to that journal for its previous publication of my work and for the support then rendered. The March number also contains Charles's translation of the second *nota preliminare* (page 223), which I had sent to Maynard, who has been an editor. Of course the victim of a piracy remains almost helpless himself.

Meanwhile several people in India were in opposition, and my old adversary Surgeon Colonel Lawrie, of Hyderabad, who was now converted to Laveranity delivered a furious attack in the *Lancet* of 3 December (the number which printed Bignami's article) and also in the Indian papers under the name of Buggobutty Bose, MD. Both articles were absurd, but they perverted many people, including even my friend Mr Reid of Nowgong. I was pummelled on one side by the pirates and on the other by the sceptics but was too exhausted to defend myself from either.*

I had seen my chief, Surgeon General Harvey, Director General IMS, when he was taking over the office from Surgeon General Cleghorn on 17 February 1898 in Calcutta. Since then he and his secretary, Surgeon Major Leslie, had been at Simla (I think that I never met the latter). They congratulated me politely when I reported my successes, but they asked no questions, never sent for me, never ordered anyone to inspect or to verify my work, never gave me any assistance (except that of a native draughtsman who was of no use), interrupted me for five months over kala-azar just at the climax of my labours, and refused to assure me that I was to be retained on malaria duty after the 17 February 1899. Owing to constant changes of station and the necessity of living in separate hotels we had spent more than £300 (about 4800 rupees) since 1895 over and above my salary,† and if I were now sent back to my regiment at Secunderabad I should have to pay the expenses of my family's journey there and next year should be obliged to go with the regiment to Burma. On 6 December I wrote to Leslie explaining all this, asking for six months' furlough to England at the end of my special duty in order to place my family there if I was to return to my regiment, and begging again for the required assurance. In reply he only told me that Dr Harvey was coming to Calcutta on the 15th. I was granted by the latter a three-minute interview in which he complimented me upon my work but refused to come to my laboratory. He allowed my leave to England but could not promise to continue me in the malaria work and struck me as being a mild but ineffectual man who took little interest in the matter. Soon, however, the confirmation of Drs Wright and Ruffer

* I was asked later which I preferred, the thieves who stole my pearls or the swine which trod them into the mire. I replied that at least the thieves knew their value. It requires some mental acuity to be a pirate, none to be a "pseudosceptic."

† This was 1000 rupees a month while I was on special duty and less on regimental duty. A friend, nine years my junior, who was one of the Calcutta medical officers was drawing 1700 rupees a month and had a lucrative private practice as well.

and of the Italians must have reached him (I sent him one of the latters' notes) and he wrote:

DIRECTOR GENERAL INDIAN MEDICAL SERVICE, CALCUTTA,
2.1.99.

MY DEAR ROSS,

I have spoken to the Government and to the Hon Member in the Home Dept. and do not think they will make any difficulty about putting you again on special duty when you return from leave. I think, therefore, you may safely apply for furlough as I know you need a rest after your hard work.

Yours sincerely,
B HARVEY.

In other words this chief of a great service entrusted with the health of three hundred millions of people was not free to continue one of his own officers in the investigation of a disease which killed over a million of those people annually without going round begging to laymen for permission.

Of course this letter was useless to me—members of council were apt to change their mind. In order to carry out the second part of my programme, the study of the local carriers of malaria in India, I should require at least five years' permanent duty there with an adequate salary and staff. It was absurd to expect such things then in India. I had to deal with an army without an intelligence department and with a general who took no interest in the enemy's movements and did not trouble to ascertain what I required. I therefore bought my passage home at once and decided to retire on reaching England.

Interleaved in my laboratory notebook there is a cutting from the *Pioneer* describing the dinner of the Indian Medical Service held at Simla on 19 September 1898.* Harvey presided and proposed "prosperity to the grand old service to which we are all proud to belong ... we shall go on doing our duty in the future as in the past (applause).... I claim for the Indian Medical Service that it rises to its duty and is true to itself on all occasions (loud applause).... I saw it stated by a correspondent in the *Pioneer* the other day—I wish people would not write to the papers—that the IMS is a decadent service. Don't you believe it, gentlemen

* On the same date we were given full military titles without the prefix "Surgeon," which many disliked.

(applause)"—and so on. If I had been present I should have applauded as loudly as anyone, but the speech was that of the colonel of a dragoon regiment rather than that of the head of a great scientific corps. There was not a word about science in it. The service had done all he claimed for it; its defect was that it had not kept pace with scientific advances in recent years. The waving of swords will not win victories and the waving of lancets and prescriptions will not maintain empires in health. Nevertheless, I thought more highly of Dr Harvey when, some time later, he came to me in Liverpool and frankly admitted the mistakes which had been made.

The truth is that of the few medical problems which have been solved most have been solved by accident or by some lucky lead in other sciences, few indeed by express intention and long effort; and when such a case occurred it met with general incredulity among the many who never "read, mark, learn, and inwardly digest." One can scarcely blame these people more than one can blame the venerable cow which impedes our motor car in the narrow country lane! She was born in the quiet fields; to her the noisy engine of progress is a thing either to be fought or to be feared; she opposes it with horns or heels or scampers foolishly before it until, escaping up some lucky bylane, she can watch it with bovine anger safely receding in the distance and so go back to her peaceful browsing!

Dr Laveran had long asked me for an account of my work for the Paris *Académie de Médecine*. My article[50] was finished on the last day of 1898* and a translation of it was presented to the *Académie* on 24 January 1899 and was reported upon by Laveran on 31 January.[57] Dr Laveran's report (which reached me later) gives me full credit and my paper repeated the acknowledgments to him and to Manson which I gave in my proteosoma report (page 162). Let me hope then that, at least, I shall never be included in the great genus Savant parasite!

Lastly, on 16 February 1899, just before leaving India, I sent to the Director General a concluding report "on the subject of the practical results as regards the prevention of the disease (malaria) which may be expected to arise from my researches." This described briefly the methods which were subsequently employed with success in West Africa, Ismailia, Havana, the Federated Malay States, Panama, and elsewhere. The article[58] was published in the *Indian Medical Gazette* for July 1899.

In those days, when an officer had been placed on special duty for any

* This was before I changed my opinion regarding the "black spores" (page 202).

purpose and his work was done, orders conveying the thanks of the government which had employed him were generally issued as some record that his duty had been faithfully performed. I was not so fortunate and from that day to this have never received any recognition that I am aware of from the Government of India or even from my old service. I have never been consulted even on my own subject by that government or by the India Office; never placed on any committee connected with it; never been asked officially for my advice; never received any Indian honour, honorary promotion, or reward. In 1912 I was advised to ask for one of the small "good service pensions" which were then sometimes given, but science evidently did not count as such and I was refused. Out of nearly 50 honours bestowed upon me by governments, universities, academies, and societies only one* has ever reached me from India; Indian writers, from G M Giles downwards, have generally attributed my work to others and, much worse than this, have obstinately opposed my methods for the reduction of malaria. In fact they have never forgiven me—for what I cannot imagine. Probably it was nothing but the sheer ineptitude of unintellectuals who "despise science," but if so the question remains whether such barbarians are fit to rule so great an empire.

My letters to Manson during this period contain chiefly brief notes about our failures, but I am glad to record, in honour of the memory of Mahomed Bux, the following from my letter of 5 January: "Mahomed Bux, however, who can make a mosquito do anything, persuades them to bite in the daytime simply by holding the test tube containing the insect against the skin of the patient." I forget who discovered this a year or two later. Let me now conclude with extracts from my two last letters of this series.

CALCUTTA,
15 *February* 1899.

DEAR DR MANSON,

Daniels went away on the 12th for Africa. Our bad luck has clung to us to the last. *Anopheles pictus* [really *A rossi*] has absolutely refused crescents and also tertian—according to a few experiments. I cannot get a single case of human malaria....

I am feeling better since my report has been finished and often feel

* The Barclay Memorial Bronze Medal, Asiatic Society, Bengal, 20 May 1903. I was made Consulting Member, Advisory Board, Indian Research Fund, but think that I have only once been consulted by it.

inclined to stay. I am leaving hosts of beautiful experiments to the Italians and others. It is a great pity but can't be helped.

We made an observation lately which throws doubt on the authenticity of the black spores—at least I think so—Daniels doesn't. I have reported to Government accordingly.

I have also reported to Government on the practical benefits likely to arise from the mosquito theory if they follow it up properly. Will show you a copy of the report....

... It would certainly be a good thing to do research in India steadily, but there are other things to be considered and many cogent reasons why I should now leave India for good. I fear also that I may even sell my microscopes. My original intention was to take my pension and adopt literature, which I know will pay me better than the microscope, though I confess that it may not be so grand a thing as research on medical subjects. Now that the great problem is solved I feel I have done my duty and may sing *nunc dimittis* and look after those essential parts of clothing, the pockets. I don't think a man can be called upon justly to give up too much for the chance of doing good research in the future.

But I think Daniels will now push on matters nicely.

It is evident that the study of malaria has now entered on the third and last phase—prevention. That is, we must find out how to exterminate the malaria-bearing species of mosquito. I shall have a great deal to tell you on this score....

We start on the 22nd and hope to arrive on about the 20th March—all the way by sea.

With kind regards,
Yours sincerely,
R Ross.

"City of Corinth,"
24 Feb. In the Hooghly.

Dear Dr Manson,

This is the last of a long series of letters to you. They began nearly four years ago.

I shall have your replies bound in a volume! The solution of the great malaria problem is history you know!

We have been two days getting out of this river, the ship being a large one, but are off at midnight. We hope to arrive on about the 22nd March....

Well, I have left many things undone which I ought to have done but congratulate myself that the task you imposed on me is finished. You must cease *rubbing the lamp* for a little at all events.

I am looking forward immensely to seeing you and I have a lot more to tell you than I have conveyed by letter. I shall concoct a full history* of the solution of the problem, after the publication of which things will take their right places. It was the *great induction* which did it—nothing else.

With kind regards,
Yours very sincerely,
RONALD ROSS.

So I said goodbye to my laboratory—the mean little building in its grove of trees; to my birds and my mosquitoes; to my faithful Mahomed Bux and my other helpers. Years later I heard that, as I wished, Mahomed had been retained by someone (? the Calcutta municipality) in employment here until he died. Whether the laboratory still exists I do not know—no one has troubled to tell me. Ah, the beautiful researches which might have been! I have them still in my mind. They have never been done. By the aid of proteosoma I had intended to work out the whole mathematical theory of parasitic infection, like Fourier's *Théorie Analytique de la Chaleur*, and then to have investigated *treatment*, not medically but scientifically. Had this been done what sums would have been saved during the war! I could go back there tomorrow (if the place still exists) and start the work again exactly as I left it 23 years ago—not biology but real measured science. But I was fated, I think, never to do any microscopical investigation again. Of course the great report on my work in July and August could never be written.

The enthusiast is rare, the successful enthusiast very rare. When he is a medical investigator he is perhaps the most valuable thing which the death-bereaved world can possess. But she does not know this and throws him away like an old shoe upon the rubbish heap. So they remain, he with his memories and she with her dead.

On the quay we said goodbye to our faithful servants Lutchman and Berlisi. We never heard of them again, though I advertised for the former in 1911.

Once more, as in 1865, I remember the brown water of the great Hooghly turning green and then blue as the *City of Corinth* panted out to the ocean. The four years were past, but the Great Problem had been solved. Now it remained only to apply the solution—to apply it *immediately*—to the saving of human life on the large scale.

* This book is the "history."

References

1 Ross R. Malaria in Greece. *Journal of Tropical Medicine*, 15 Nov 1906, and University Review, May 1907. Various studies; and suggests that the decadence of Greece might have been partly due to the entry of malaria from Asia and Africa. Also *The Times*, 11 Oct 1906, and *Smithsonian Report*, Washington DC, 1908.

2 Jones WHS. *Malaria and Greek history*. University Press, Manchester, 1909, 175 pages. A scholarly analysis of the subject.

3 Ross R with 20 collaborators for special sections. *The prevention of malaria*. J Murray, London, Sept 1910. 2nd ed, June 1911, with mathematical addendum on the theory of happenings, 711 pages.

4 Varro MT (116–28 BC). *Rerum rusticarum*, Lib I. Says that in marshes there are animals which are too small to be seen but which enter the mouth and nostrils and cause troublesome disease.

5 Palladius RTA (4th century AD). *De re rustica*, Lib I. Connects marshes with pestilence and inimical animals.

6 Lancisi JM. *De noxiis paludum effluviis, eorumque remediis*, Roma 1717. Repeats the same conjectures, studies mosquitoes, and advocates drainage against malaria.

7 Meckel H. *Allgemeine Zeitschrift für Psychiatrie*, 1847. Discovers the malarial pigment.

8 Laveran A. *Bulletin de l'Académie de Médicine (Paris)*, 23 Nov 1880. Discovers the parasites of malaria.

9 Manson P. Linnean Society 1878 and Pathological Society 1881. Describes partially the development of *Filaria bancrofti* in certain mosquitoes.

10 Smith T, Kilborne FL. The nature, causation and prevention of Texas or southern cattle fever. Bureau of Animal Industry, *Department of Agriculture Bulletin I*, Washington DC, 1893.

11 Bruce D. Reports on tsetse fly disease or nagana in Zululand: Ubombo, Dec 1895 and May 1896. Proves that the disease is caused by a trypanosome which is carried mechanically by the tsetse fly *Glossina palpalis*.

12 Nuttall GHF. On the role of insects... as carriers... of diseases of men and animals: *Johns Hopkins Hospital Reports*, VIII, and *Hygienische Rundschau*, 1899. Also eight

papers on the mosquito-malaria theory: *Zentralblatt für Bakteriologie*, 1899. History of the subject.
13 Beauperthuy LD. *Gaceta Official de Cumaná*, Venezuela, 23 May 1854. Conjectured that malaria might be produced by the poison of mosquitoes injected under the skin when they bite us.
14 Finlay C. *Anales de la Real Academia de Ciencias*, 14 August 1881. Conjectures that mosquitoes carry yellow fever by their bites from the sick to the healthy.
15 King AFA. Insects and disease – mosquitoes and malaria. *Popular Science Monthly*, New York, Sept 1883. Conjectures that mosquitoes carry malaria from marshes to men and gives nineteen reasons for this supposition.
16 Laveran A. *Traité des fièvres palustres*. Doin, Paris 1884. Conjectures (page 457) that mosquitoes may play the same role in malaria as in filariasis.
17 Ross R. *Researches on malaria; being the Nobel Medical Prize Lecture delivered at Stockholm*, 12 *Dec* 1902. PA Norstedt, Stockholm, and *Journal of the Royal Army Medical Corps*, April, May, June 1905. History of researches up to 1902, with bibliography and plates of 25. Translation into German by Dr C Schilling (G Fischer in Jena 1905) and Italian by F Maiocco (Lib Editrice Universitaria, Torino 1905).
18 Ross R. Fever with intestinal lesions: South Indian Branch, British Medical Association 1892. Cases of febricula with abdominal tenderness; enteroseptic fevers; a study of Indian fevers; all in *Indian Medical Gazette* 1892. Conjectures that malarial fevers, or at least many fevers, may be due to intestinal sepsis.
19 Ross R. Some observations on haematozoic theories of malaria. *Medical Reporter* (afterwards *Indian Lancet*), 1893. Nodulated and vacuolated corpuscles and the solution of corpuscles mistaken for parasites. *Indian Medical Record* 1893. The third element of the blood and the malaria parasite and a list of natural appearances in the blood which have been mistaken for forms of the malaria parasite. *Indian Medical Gazette* 1894. Shows that various objects described by writers in India as plasmodia are only artifacts and criticises the accepted epidemiology of malaria.
20 Manson P. On the nature and significance of the crescentic and flagellated bodies in malarial blood. *British Medical Journal* 8 Dec 1894. Conjectures that these forms of the plasmodium are intended to infect mosquitoes of "a similar suctorial insect" and that the "free flagella" are flagellated spores.
21 Ficalbi E. Revisione systematica d fam delle Culicidae europea, Florence 1896.
22 Ross R. Parkes Memorial Prize Essay on Malaria. Army Medical School, Netley, March 1895 (unpublished). Analyses the accepted epidemiology of malaria.
23 Ross R, Salvin-Moore JE, Walker CE. A new microscopical diagnostic method etc. *Lancet*, 27 July 1907. And on the existence of centrosomes... in red blood corpuscles of vertebrates. Pathological Society of London, vol 58, part I, 1907.
24 Ross R. Observations on the crescent-sphere-flagella metamorphosis of the malaria parasite within the mosquito: South Indian Branch, British Medical Association, 17 Dec 1895, and *Indian Lancet* 1896.
25 Ross R. Papers on the thick-film process for malaria diagnosis. *Lancet*, 10 Jan, *Journal of Tropical Medicine*, 2 Feb, and *Thompson Yates and Johnston Laboratories Reports*, vol V, part I, 1903.
26 Ross R. *Report on the cultivation of proteosoma, Labbé, in grey mosquitoes*: Government

Printing, Calcutta, dated 21 May 1898, circulated privately but not allowed to be issued till Oct 1898; second edition (many printers' errors), 1901. Describes cultivation of a plasmodium of birds in *Culex fatigans* up to the maturity of zygotes, with complete differential proofs, technique, and nine plates. Reprinted in *Indian Medical Gazette*, Nov and Dec 1898.

27 Ross R. Surg Lt Col Lawrie and the parasite of malaria. *Indian Lancet*, 1 Oct 1896. Polemic against a sceptic.

28 Ross R. Some experiments in the production of malarial fever by means of the mosquito. South Indian Branch, British Medical Association Dec 1896 (read 30 Oct) and *Indian Medical Gazette*, 1897. Failure to infect men by drinking water and by mosquito bites.

29 Manson P. The life history of the malaria germ outside the human body: Goulstonian Lectures. *British Medical Journal* 15, 21, 28 March 1896. Elaborates his mosquito theory, conjectures that plasmodia are parasites of mosquitoes independent of men, infecting men through water or dust, and quotes Ross's recent work at length in support of his views.

30 Bignami A. Policlinico, Rome, 15 July 1896 and translation, *Lancet* ii p 1363 Nov 14, p 1441 Nov 21; 1896. Rejects Manson's theory because (he says) the flagellate bodies are dying forms but conjectures that mosquitoes bring malaria from marshes to men (as King suggested in 15).

31 Sakharoff N. Centr f Bakter 1894–5. Describes the chromatin in the plasmodia, including the alleged "flagella."

32 Ross R. On a condition necessary to the transformation of the malaria crescent. *British Medical Journal*, 30 Jan 1897. Further observations on the transformation of crescents: South Indian Branch, British Medical Association, July 1897, and *Indian Medical Gazette*, Jan 1898. Disproves Bignami's contention in 30.

33 Bignami A. Come si prendone le febre malariche: richeriche sperimentali: *Bollettino e atti della Accademia Medica di Roma*, dated 15 Nov; trans *Lancet*, 3 and 10 Dec 1898. Records the alleged infection of the man Sola by the bites of mosquitoes on 1 Nov and further experiments.

34 Ross R. Notes on some cases of malaria, *Amoeba coli*, and Cercomonas. *Indian Medical Gazette*, May 1897.

35 MacCallum WG. *Lancet*, 13 Nov 1897 and *Journal of Experimental Medicine*, 1898, III, no. I. Proves the same thing in the plasmodia.

36 Simond PD. *Annales de l'Institut Pasteur*, July 1897. Shows that the "flagellate forms" of *Coccidium oviforme* are really sperms.

37 Ross R. The principle of repeated medication for curing infections. *British Medical Journal*, 2 July 1921. Argues that as one dose of a remedy can destroy only a percentage of the invading organisms the doses must be repeated to effect extirpation and gives a formula for the number of times.

38 Ross R. Report on a preliminary investigation into malaria in the Sigur Ghat, Ootacamund: South Indian Branch, British Medical Association, Feb 1898, and *Indian Medical Gazette*, April 1898. Researches done in 1897 before those of 42 and 43.

39 Ross R. Parasite of mosquitoes found in India between 1895 and 1899. *Journal of Hygiene*, Cambridge, April 1906.

40 The Indian shepherds; a fragment. *English Review*, Sept 1913, 7 pages. Verses commenced in 1898.

41 *Philosophies*. Murray, 1910; subsequent editions in 1910, 1911; 56 pages. Verses written 1881–99.

42 Ross R. On some peculiar pigmented cells found in two mosquitoes fed on malarial blood, with notes by J Smyth, P Manson, Bland Sutton, and Dr Thin and a drawing by P Manson. *British Medical Journal*, 18 Dec 1897. Discovers *Plasmodium falciparum* in two *Anopheles* (unmistakably described—probably *A stephensi*), after many failures with species of *Stegomyia* and *Culex*.

43 Ross R. Pigmented cells in mosquitoes. *British Medical Journal*, 26 Feb 1898. The same cells found in two more mosquitoes and answers to objections.

44 Giles GM. *Handbook of gnats or mosquitoes*: J Bale, Sons and Danielsson, London, Feb 1900; 2nd ed Feb 1902.

45 Manson P. Surgeon Major Ronald Ross's recent investigation on the mosquito malaria theory. *British Medical Journal*, 18 June 1898. Gives the same information derived from 26 and from Ross's letters (one serious error regarding halteridium), with three figures and notes accepting the discovery by Laveran, Metchnikoff, and Nuttall.

46 Manson P. The mosquito and the malaria parasite: read at the annual meeting of the British Medical Association at Edinburgh on the 28th July 1898; *Lancet* (with one figure), 20th Aug; *Journal of Tropical Medicine* (one figure), Aug; *British Medical Journal* (one full page and two other figures) complete, 24 Sept 1898. Describes the full life-cycle of Proteosoma (and therefore presumably of all the *Plasmodia*) in mosquitoes, with the collection of the protospores in the salivary glands and the experimental infection of healthy birds, communicated by R Ross in letters and telegram.

47 Ross R. *Malarial fever, its cause, prevention, and treatment*: University Press, Liverpool, February 1902, 68 pages. Enlarged edition of 48. Translated into German (Wilhelm Süsserott, Berlin 1904) and into modern Greek (Ethnikoy Typographeioy, Athens 1906).

48 Anonymous (R Ross). *Instructions for the prevention of malarial fever*: University Press, Liverpool, 1899. Popular exposition of 14 pages for residents in malarious places. Sixth edition in 1901.

49 Ross R. *Preliminary report on the infection of birds with proteosoma by the bites of mosquitoes*: Government Press, Calcutta, dated 11 Oct 1898; also *Indian Medical Gazette*, Jan 1899, and *British Medical Journal*, with additions 18 Feb 1899. Delayed information already partly given by Manson in 46 from Ross's work done in July and August 1898.

50 Ross R. Du rôle des moustiques dans le paludisme: *Bulletin de l'Académie de Médecine (Paris)*, 24 Jan, and *Annales de l'Institut Pasteur*, 1899, p 136. Summarises his work.

51 Ross R. On the newly discovered Leishman-Donovan parasites. *British Medical Journal*, 14, 21, and 28 Nov, and *Thompson Yates and Johnston Laboratories Reports*, vol V, part II, 1903.

52 Ross R. Report on Kala-Azar: dated 30 Jan 1899, Government Press, Calcutta. Many notes on malaria.

53 Koch R. Ueber die Entwickelung der Malaria Parasiten: *Zeitschrift für Hygiene und Infektionskrankheiten*, Bd XXXII, 1899. Confirms Ross's work and adjudicates on the history.

54 Grassi B. La malaria propagata per mezzo de peculiare insetti. *Atti della R Accademia nazionale dei Lincei*, seduta del 6 Nov 1898.The same as above with further vague epidemiological reasons.

55 Bastianelli G, Bignami A, Grassi B. Coltivazione d semilune malariche dell' uomo nell' *Anopheles claviger* Fabr. *Atti della R Accademia nazionale dei Lincei*, seduta del 4 Dec 1898. Find zygotes in two *A claviger* apparently fed on cases of malaria, but give no details and no proofs. The authors think that Ross's mosquitoes of 42 were of this species but render false accounts of his experiments.

56 Bastianelli G, Bignami A, Grassi B. Ulteriori ricerche sul ciclo parassiti malarici umani nel corpo del zanzarone. *Att dell R Accademia nazionale dei Lincei*, seduta del 8 Jan 1899. Find Ross's cycle in other *A claviger* but give no details and no proofs and small acknowledgements. Subsequent papers by the same authors at sitting of 5 Feb and 7 May 1899 or elsewhere, jointly or severally, incriminate two other species of Italian anopheles, both for *P falciparum* and *P vivax*, and describe and figure the cytology of the cycle.

57 Laveran A. Sur un Travail de M le Dr Ronald Ross, etc: *Bulletin de l'Académie de Médecine*, séance du 31 Jan 1899. Adjudicates on the history of the subject.

58 Ross R. Letter to government of India on malaria prevention by means of mosquito reduction, dated 16 Feb 1899: *Indian Medical Gazette* (with Editor's title), July 1899. Outlines mosquito-reduction as a public-health measure for appropriate localities.

This edition of
The Great Malaria Problem and its Solution
consists of 300 numbered copies published by
the Keynes Press, London.
It has been designed by Sebastian Carter
and set, in Baskerville,
printed, and bound by
Cambridge University Press
on a cream laid paper.

This copy is No. 36.

The Keynes Press emblem
is a profile of Sir Geoffrey Keynes
engraved by David Gentleman
and based on the bust by Nigel Boonham
in the National Portrait Gallery